Study Guide to Accompany

Mohr: Johnson's Psychiatric-Mental Health Nursing

FIFTH EDITION

Carol J. Cornwell, PhD, RN, CS

Assistant Professor of Nursing
Director, Center for Nursing Scholarship
ANA Certified Adult Psychiatric Mental Health
Clinical Nursing Specialist
Georgia Southern University
Statesboro, Georgia

Visit the Lippincott Williams & Wilkins Website
http://www.lww.com

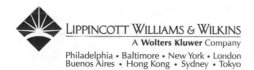

LIPPINCOTT WILLIAMS & WILKINS
A **Wolters Kluwer** Company

Philadelphia • Baltimore • New York • London
Buenos Aires • Hong Kong • Sydney • Tokyo

ging Editor: Doris S. Wray
r Production Editor: Rosanne Hallowell
ior Production Manager: Helen Ewan
anaging Editor / Production: Erika Kors
Manufacturing Manager: William Alberti
Compositor: Lippincott Williams & Wilkins
Printer: Victor Graphics

9 8 7 6 5 4 3 2 1

ISBN 0-7817-4021-5

Care has been taken to confirm the accuracy of the information presented and to describe generally accepted practices. However, the author, editors, and publisher are not responsible for errors or omissions or for any consequences from application of the information in this book and make no warranty, express or implied, with respect to the content of the publication.

The author, editors, and publisher have exerted every effort to ensure that drug selection and dosage set forth in this text are in accordance with the current recommendations and practice at the time of publication. However, in view of ongoing research, changes in government regulations, and the constant flow of information relating to drug therapy and drug reactions, the reader is urged to check the package insert for each drug for any change in indications and dosage and for added warnings and precautions This is particularly important when the recommended agent is a new or infrequently employed drug.

Some drugs and medical devices presented in this publication have Food and Drug Administration (FDA) clearance for limited use in restricted research settings. It is the responsibility of the health care provider to ascertain the FDA status of each drug or device planned for use in his or her clinical practice.

LWW.com

To the Student

Psychiatric–Mental Health Nursing is perhaps the only nursing specialty area that is truly "cross discipline"—psychiatric nursing concepts apply to all clinical specialties in nursing. Concepts and understandings that you will gain in psychiatric nursing will be useful to you as you enter the working world, and begin to understand just how many biopsychological issues are operating in each and every client with whom you will work. Many students who have found positions in medical-surgical, pediatric, ICU, and other clinical areas of the hospital return to their nursing program faculty and comment, "I never knew how much psych I'd need to use on this unit! . . . I wish I had taken it more seriously!" The things you will learn in this important course will help you in working with clients and families in all areas of nursing. So take it seriously, try to learn all you can, and remember the concepts and interventions you will learn in psychiatric nursing, because they will be invaluable to you as an RN.

This *Study Guide to Accompany Mohr: Johnson's Psychiatric–Mental Health Nursing, 5th edition*, is designed to be used with your textbook to help you incorporate knowledge that you learn in the classroom, through reading, and in the clinical setting. This combination of information sources will help you develop strategies to answer questions that will arise in the "real world." It is recommended that you use this Study Guide on a regular basis, completing chapter exercises prior to the corresponding classroom lecture. The Guide will help you pull concepts from the textbook, and will also challenge you to think about ways in which you can use your new knowledge.

In Chapters 1 to 17, the questions in the Study Guide include matching, multiple choice, NCLEX-style exam questions, and a number of case studies, diagrams, and personal reflection exercises. From Chapters 18 to 30, the Guide is organized slightly differently. Each of the chapter exercises revolves around a clinical Case Study scenario. Data are presented for each clinical story, and questions are asked along the way. By the time you complete the Case Study Exercises for each chapter, you will have a solid knowledge base for dealing therapeutically with various client behaviors, recognizing signs and symptoms of the most common psychiatric disorders, understanding treatment, and implementing nursing interventions, including developing plans of care. You aren't given the answers for the Case Study Exercises; therefore, you'll need to read your text, talk with peers, and use your developing clinical knowledge in order to arrive at the most therapeutic answers throughout each Case Study.

I hope the Study Guide will help you to analyze and solidify your learning, as well as assist you to become an astute critical thinker. I welcome general and specific comments and suggestions about this Study Guide from students like you. Please e-mail me if you have any ideas. Best wishes as you embark on your journey into Psychiatric–Mental Health Nursing!

Carol Cornwell, PhD, MS, CS
Email: ccornwel@gasou.edu

To Faculty

This *Study Guide to Accompany Mohr: Johnson's Psychiatric–Mental Health Nursing, 5th edition*, was designed using some familiar elements (such as matching and multiple choice), as well as a unique new format for clinical Case Studies.

In the first half of the Study Guide (Chapters 1–17), I have incorporated a number of exercises that will help students solidify and learn concepts and principles; this section also includes diagrams and care plans in selected situations.

In the second half of the Study Guide (Chapters 18–30), each chapter is organized around a clinical Case Study, which is presented in parts. The client admission information is identified, and the student is taken through a clinical scenario that reflects major concepts and clinical information that are critical for caring for the client. For each point at which data are added to the scenario, a series of questions are asked of the student. Each Case Study also includes a Nursing Care Plan (Nursing Process Worksheet) for students to complete to target specific problematic behaviors. These chapters were designed to be useful to faculty as well as students. Perhaps Study Guide exercises can be done as either pre-class assignments, or even in the classroom. Students could be assigned into groups and present the Case Study in parts, answering appropriate questions. You could also modify or add to the clinical data presented in order to illustrate specific content that you might wish to highlight. Answers are not provided for the Case Study Exercises; students will need to explore their text, talk with peers, and use clinical knowledge in order to arrive at the most therapeutic answers throughout each Case Study.

I am hopeful that the Case Study approach will help the student to think critically instead of answering rote questions. I am very open to suggestions and ideas that you may have regarding the content of the Study Guide; e-mails are welcome. Please let me know if this Guide meets your needs and if there are ways in which it could be enhanced to augment your classroom teaching.

Carol Cornwell, PhD, MS, CS
Email: ccornwel@gasou.edu

Contents

UNIT V
Nursing Care for Special Populations

Answer Key

Introduction to Psychiatric–Mental Health Nursing

Chapter 1 introduces the concepts of mental health and mental illness. The significance of mental health issues in America is highlighted, including trends, problems, and goals related to the delivery of mental health care and the treatment of mental illness. The role of various organizations in promoting mental health awareness is discussed. In addition, the role of psychiatric–mental health nurses, including levels of practice and associated responsibilities in psychiatric mental health care, are outlined.

OBJECTIVES

When you have completed the exercises in this chapter, you will be able to:

- Define mental health and mental illness.

- Describe the five Axes and diagnoses that appear on each, in the multiaxial diagnostic system used in the *Diagnostic and Statistical Manual of Mental Disorders*, 4th edition, text revision (DSM-IV-TR).

- Define terminology used in psychiatric–mental health care.

- Apply the principles guiding psychiatric nursing to a clinical example.

- Describe feelings and thoughts associated with beginning in psychiatric–mental health clinical practice.

- Discuss and develop suggestions for self-growth and awareness in psychiatric–mental health.

KEY TERMS

Altruism: The desire to contribute something valuable to society.

Culturally competent care: Care provided in a manner acceptable to a client's cultural background, regardless of whether the health care professional who delivers the care is from the same ethnic or minority group as the client.

Dual diagnosis: Diagnosis of both a mental disorder and a co-occurring substance abuse problem.

Horizontal violence: Anger or negativity a nurse directs toward another nurse.

Medication adherence: The actual taking of medications as prescribed; also called *medication compliance*.

Mental disorders: Health conditions marked by alterations in thinking, mood, or behavior that cause distress, impair ability to function, or both.

Mental health: The successful performance of mental function, resulting in productive activities, fulfilling relationships, and the ability to adapt to change and cope with adversity.

Mental health nursing: The care of well and at-risk populations to prevent mental illness or provide immediate treatment for those with early signs of a psychiatric disorder.

Mental illness: A clinically significant behavioral or psychological syndrome experienced by a person and marked by distress, disability, or the risk of suffering, disability, or loss of freedom.

Psychiatric–mental health nursing: The diagnosis and treatment of human responses to actual or potential mental health problems.

Psychiatric nursing: The care and rehabilitation of people with identifiable mental illnesses or disorders.

Tautology: A logical error in reasoning.

Chapter Outline

MENTAL HEALTH AND MENTAL ILLNESS
The Mental Health–Illness Continuum
Mental Health: A Report of the Surgeon General
Elements of Mental Health
Influences on Mental Health
Incidence and Prevalence of Mental Illness
Etiology of Mental Illness
Diagnosis of Mental Illness
Prevention and Treatment of Mental Illness
Problems in Treating Mental Illness
   Cost-Related Issues
   Stigma

Revolving Door Treatment
Lack of Parity
Limited Access to Services
Goals of Care and Methods of Achievement
Beyond Response to Recovery
Reintegration into Society
Mental Health Parity
Culturally Competent Care
Medication Adherence
Self-Help Movements and Advocacy
National Alliance for the Mentally Ill
Family Advocacy Movement
Psychiatric Advance Directives
PSYCHIATRIC–MENTAL HEALTH NURSING
Nursing Process and Standards of Care
Levels of Practice
Guiding Principles
The Role of the Psychiatric Nurse as a Team Member
Learning to Provide Appropriate Care
Understanding the Client's View of Mental Health Care
Managing Stress and Burnout

KEY TOPICS

Mental health and mental illness: elements, influences, demographics, etiology, and diagnoses of mental illness.

Preventing and treating mental illness: problems (cost, stigma, limitations in access); goals and the processes of mental health care delivery (reintegration into society, mental health parity, cultural issues, medication adherence); self-help movements and advocacy.

Psychiatric–mental health nursing: Standards of Care; levels of practice and guidelines; role of the psychiatric nurse as team member.

■ Exercises

MATCHING

General Matching

Match the term in Part A with the statement that applies to the term in Part B:

PART A

a. Mental illness
b. Dual diagnosis
c. Multi-axial system in psychiatry
d. Tautology
e. Stigma
f. Parity

g. Adherence
h. NAMI
i. Horizontal violence
j. Altruism

PART B

1. _____ "I am a psychiatric nurse because I want to contribute to society."
2. _____ A system of diagnosis in psychiatry in which five axes represent a holistic view of the person and his/her difficulties
3. _____ When a person is suffering from both a mental disorder and also a substance abuse problem
4. _____ When a client does what has been suggested in order to get better
5. _____ Clinically significant syndrome experienced by a person; marked by functional disturbance, including distress, disability, or the risk of suffering or loss of freedom
6. _____ A sign of job-related stress and burnout; when nurses act angrily toward each other
7. _____ "He acts like a schizophrenic because he has schizophrenia."
8. _____ An important national self-help group developed to increase public awareness, family support, research, and education about mental illnesses
9. _____ When society labels or blames the mentally ill individual for his/her problems
10. _____ Equality

DSM-IV-TR Matching

The following exercise is designed to help familiarize you with the DSM-IV-TR multi-axial system of diagnosis in psychiatry. Match the clinical issue with the Axis on which it would be diagnosed (you may use the Axes more than once):

a. _____ Hypertension
b. _____ Schizophrenia
c. _____ Mental retardation
d. _____ Borderline personality disorder
e. _____ Extremely stressful 6 months, with loss of mother and fire in home

f. _____ Functioning at a moderate
level: 75

g. _____ Dementia: Alzheimer's

h. _____ Alcohol withdrawal syndrome

1. Axis I
2. Axis II
3. Axis III
4. Axis IV
5. Axis V

COMPLETION

Complete each sentence with the appropriate content:

1. Psychiatric–mental health nurses work in environments that are very stressful and must be aware of _____ behaviors such as calling in sick, dawdling, or intentionally forgetting things.

2. Jane has decided to go into psychiatric–mental health nursing because she is very _____ and wants to contribute something important to society.

3. _____ is the ninth leading cause of death in the United States.

4. Juan has told his psychiatric nurse that he needs to pray before each meal, and since the nurse is _____, she includes Juan's daily prayers into his care plan.

5. At the _____ level of practice, psychiatric–mental health nurses promote and encourage the maintenance of health and prevention of disorder, assess biopsychosocial functioning, are case managers, and promote self-care activities.

CASE STUDY

You are working with Ketreshia, a 28-year-old African-American woman who was admitted to your psychiatric unit 2 hours ago with the diagnosis of paranoid schizophrenia. She came into the emergency department last night after being found in a parking lot, partially dressed, yelling and screaming that "the devil is out tonight, and no one is safe from his wrath!" Since admission, she has been given medications to help with her thoughts and has calmed down a great deal. You are new on this unit and you are assigned to care for Ketreshia. When you approach her, you notice that she is disheveled and smells of alcohol. You ask her how she is doing right now, and she seems to ignore you, gets up, and walks away from you.

1. Pretend for a moment that you are Ketreshia. Close your eyes, and try to imagine yourself in the situation described above.
   a. List some of the thoughts you might be having.
   b. List some emotional feelings that you could imagine having.
   c. Try and imagine what you would want your nurse to say or do.

2. As a student, put yourself into this situation and imagine how you would feel. List some of the first thoughts and feelings that come into your mind.

3. Discuss some of the things that our society would think and believe about Ketreshia's behavior. Would stigma and stereotyping be a part of these beliefs? If so, how?

4. With what you are learning about your role as a psychiatric–mental health nurse, list six guiding principles and beliefs about Ketreshia and the care that she deserves that would guide your view of her nursing care:
   a. _____
   b. _____
   c. _____
   d. _____
   e. _____
   f. _____

5. The following are common fears or thoughts that a new psychiatric–mental health nurse or a nursing student might feel when assigned to care for Ketreshia. For each one listed, write down a

suggestion or a thought to remember that might help you deal with your concern:

a. Why did Ketreshia walk away when I asked her a therapeutic question?

b. Will my attempts at intervening with Ketreshia ever produce a therapeutic effect?

c. What will I talk about with Ketreshia?

d. What if Ketreshia doesn't get well?

CRITICAL THINKING AND SELF-EVALUATION

Think about a time in your life when you saw or heard of a person who had some type of mental illness. It may have been in school, in your family, on television, or in a movie.

1. What are some of the ways you thought and felt about this person?

2. Do you think that your experience with mental illness in the past will have an impact on how you feel about your current psychiatric–mental health nursing course and clinical? How so?

3. Write down some of the strategies you might use to increase your awareness about your own thoughts or feelings about mental health and mental illness during this course experience.

■ NCLEX-Style Exam Questions

1. A key element in the definition of mental illness is that:

a. the individual must need medications in order for the diagnosis to be of mental origin.

b. the individual must have difficulties in functioning that cause distress and/or impairment of some type.

c. the individual must acknowledge that he or she is having difficulties in functioning.

d. the individual must have physiological symptoms that match with behaviors that are impaired.

2. In *Mental Health: A Report of the Surgeon General* (1999), all but which of the following messages were addressed?

a. Mental disorders are real health conditions.

b. Effective treatments for mental disorders are available.

c. The cost for mental health care is exorbitant and often unrealistic.

d. People with mental disorders should seek treatment.

3. All but which of the following are elements that are part of the notion of mental health?

a. Self-governance, tolerance of uncertainty

b. Reality orientation and mastery of the environment

c. Stress management and self-esteem

d. Reading, writing, and speaking ability

4. In any given year, how many people in the United States have a diagnosable mental disorder or illness?

a. 48 million

b. 100 million

c. 1 billion

d. 750,000

5. Why is depression in older adults often undiagnosed and untreated?

a. Older adults do not enter the health care system as much as younger adults.

b. Older adult depression is often seen as "normal aging."

c. Older adults are less likely to express their sadness.

d. Older adults usually die prior to the onset of depression.

6. A client with diabetes is also suffering from depression related to his diagnosis. How would the multi-axial system be applied to this client?

a. Diabetes would be diagnosed on Axis III, depression on Axis I.

b. Depression would be diagnosed on Axis I, but diabetes is not diagnosed in psychiatry.

c. Diabetes would appear on Axis II, depression on Axis III.

d. Diabetes and depression would both be diagnosed on Axis II as a dual diagnosis.

7. Newer psychotropic medications are often more effective and safer than are older medications; however, they are often more costly. Which of the following is the biggest barrier to individuals' receiving newer, more effective medication?

a. These medications are not available because they are in such great demand.

b. These medications are often not covered by the managed care system because they are expensive.

c. These medications are paid for by all insurance companies, but clients do not like to take psychotropics.

d. The side effects of newer medications are often too severe for clients to consider taking them.

8. Medical insurance coverage for medical illnesses is greater than for psychiatric illnesses. This prohibits many individuals who need psychiatric care from receiving it. The term that best describes this situation is:

a. Stigmatism related to medical coverage

b. Lack of parity

c. Limited access to services

d. Medical noncompliance

9. One of the most important factors that affects client compliance or adherence with psychotropic medications is:

a. Receiving education and information about the medication

b. A history of taking these types of medications

c. The number of other medications the client is taking

d. The support the client has at home for taking his/her medications

10. In psychiatric advance directives, clients formally declare their treatment wishes should they become ill, including the following types of interventions:

a. Where their children should be placed

b. Use of psychotropic medications, seclusion, restraint, or ECT

c. Use of life-saving devices, such as ventilators

d. Use of emergency medical technicians or ambulance services

Neuroscience: Biology and Behavior

Chapter 2 provides a basic overview of the function and structure of the nervous system, including individual neurons and neurotransmitters as well as brain regions that are organized from simpler to more complex areas. The brain's nervous tissues have the property of plasticity, which enables the brain to shape or mold itself as a result of experience. Plasticity is key to understanding why and how learning influences brain and behavior. Genetics plays a critical role in the understanding of the etiology and expression of psychiatric illnesses, although research in this area is in its infancy. The brain is the organ of the mind, and regulates all behaviors of the body. As such, it is important for psychiatric–mental health nurses to learn and understand the structure and functions of the brain and how they relate to human behavior.

LEARNING OBJECTIVES

After completing the exercises in this workbook, and studying the corresponding chapter in the textbook, the student will be able to:

- List the major structures of the brain and how they are related to behavior.

- Explain the relationship between the brain, its chemistry, and mental illness.

- Identify the basic structures of a neuron.

- Describe the process of neurotransmission.

- Discuss the concept of neuroplasticity and how it relates to mental health and mental illness.

- Briefly explain the importance of interaction between genes and environment.

- Identify neuroimaging techniques, and discuss their relative advantages and disadvantages.

- Discuss how environment can influence the course of the developing brain.

- Explain the different kinds of memory.

- Discuss the relationship between neurotransmitters and mental illness.

KEY TERMS

Action potential: The change in electrical potential on the surface of a nerve or muscle cell, often initiated by a change in cellular ionic balance.

Adaptive plasticity: An irreversible change in nervous tissue that usually affects the expression of a genotype into a phenotype.

Axon: A cylindrical neuron structure that relays information away from the cell body.

Blood-brain barrier: A protective system in the lining of blood vessels composed of endothelial cells with tight junctions, thus limiting access of blood constituents to the central nervous system.

Circadian rhythm: A rhythmic activity cycle lasting approximately 24 hours.

Critical periods: Periods during which children should be most exposed to certain stimuli for optimal development to take place. These periods vary according to different domains of functioning.

Concordance rate: The rate at which a trait expressed in one twin is expressed in another.

Dendrites: Branched processes that extend from and relay information to the cell body and receive signals from numerous neurons.

First messengers: Neurotransmitters that are responsible for transmitting impulses between nerve cells.

Glial cells: In the nervous system, non-neural cells that serve supporting and nutritive roles for neurons.

Learning: A process that occurs when organisms take in and store information as a function of experience.

Memory: Information that is stored as a result of learning.

Neurons: Nerve cells; the fundamental units of the nervous system.

Neuropeptides: The newest class of neurotransmitters, which includes endorphins and enkephalins, vasoactive intestinal peptide, cholecystokinin, and substance P.

Neuroplasticity: The ability of nervous tissue to change in its structure and functioning.

Neurotransmitters: Chemical substances that relay messages between presynaptic and postsynaptic cells and are synthesized, stored, and released by neurons.

Psychoneuroimmunology: An emerging field that focuses on the links between a person's emotions, the functioning of his or her immune system, and how both factors alter central nervous system functioning.

Reactive plasticity: A rapid, usually reversible, functional change in nervous tissue.

Receptor: A component of the cell membrane with the capacity to bind to a specific neurotransmitter.

Reuptake: The process of the terminal of a presynaptic nerve cell taking back released neurotransmitter molecules for storage and subsequent release.

Second hit: Environmental factors hypothesized to contribute to the expression and characteristics of a person's illness.

Second messengers: Secondary chemicals produced by the binding of a neurotransmitter to a receptor coupled with a G protein.

Synapse: The area involving the membrane of a presynaptic neuron (sender), the synaptic cleft, and the membrane of the postsynaptic neuron (receiver), across which a nerve impulse passes.

Synaptic cleft: A gap between the cellular membranes of the terminal of the presynaptic neuron and dendritic processes of the postsynaptic neuron.

Transcription: Process whereby a DNA sequence is copied onto RNA.

Translation: Process by which information in RNA produces amino acids (which make up proteins).

Chapter Outline

NEUROANATOMY AND NEUROPHYSIOLOGY
Neurons
Neurotransmission
Plasticity
Central Nervous System
Spinal Cord
The Brain
  Organization and Structure
    Cerebrum
    Diencephalon
    Cerebellum
    Brain Stem
    Limbic System
    Basal Ganglia

Brain Development
Neuroplasticity
The Role of Genetics
Genetics and Psychiatric Disorders
Interaction Between Genes and Environment
OTHER TOPICS IN NEUROSCIENCE
Memory, Repetition, and Learning
Circadian Rhythm
Psychoneuroimmunology
Neuroimaging Techniques

KEY TOPICS

Neuroanatomy and neurophysiology: Neurons (structure, function, cellular components); neurotransmission (neurotransmitters, receptors, first and second messengers); plasticity (nervous tissue changing structure and function).

Nervous system: central nervous system (spinal cord and brain—major structures include cerebrum, thalamus, hypothalamus, cerebellum, brainstem, limbic system, ventricles); peripheral nervous system (neurons outside the CNS); plasticity (brain's ability to develop and change).

Genetic links to mental illness: Gene structure, function, and reproduction; genetics and psychiatric disorders; gene and environment interactions.

Other neuroscience topics: Memory, repetition, learning, circadian rhythm, psychoneuroimmunology, neuroimaging techniques

■ Exercises

MATCHING

Match the term in Part A with the statement that most accurately applies to the term in Part B:

PART A

a. glial cells, neurons

b. dendrite, synapse, axon, cell body

c. Broca's and Wernicke's areas

d. cerebellum

e. neurotransmitters

f. diencephalon

g. cerebrum

h. first and second messengers

i. second hits

j. hippocampus

PART B

1. _____ In occipital lobe of brain; related to language

2. _____ Environmental vulnerability factors that come into play in contributing to problems in an already genetically predisposed individual

3. _____ Broad classes of cells in the nervous system

4. _____ Contains the thalamus, hypothalamus, and pineal gland

5. _____ Guides movement and regulates muscle tone

6. _____ Parts of neuron

7. _____ Molecules released when receptors are activated, and that exchange information between (outside the cell) and within (inside the cell) neurons

8. _____ Contains frontal, parietal, occipital, and temporal regions

9. _____ Act on receptors to transmit messages; are synthesized and stored in terminal button of neuron; and play roles in many psychiatric disorders

10. _____ when damaged, individuals cannot form new memories (called Korsakoff's syndrome)

SHORT ANSWER

1. A _____ might be the presence of experiences that are toxic, such as physical or sexual abuse, or living in a war zone when one is already genetically predisposed to mental illness.

2. _____ is the process occurring when a person takes in information as a function of experience; and _____ is the information that is stored as a result of this process.

3. The process of awakening in the morning and sleeping at nightfall, thus functioning on an approximate 24-hour cycle, is called _____.

4. _____ is the study of connections between the central nervous system, endocrine, and immune systems and how these systems interact to have an effect on health.

5. It is important to know about _____, because many medications used in psychiatry work to increase or decrease their levels in the brain.

6. The _____ includes the pons, medulla oblongata, reticular formation, and midbrain; these brain structures control many of the functions that are vital to life, such as _____, _____, _____, and _____.

7. A child must be exposed to visual input while the visual system is organizing, a developmental time that is referred to as a _____.

8. _____ plasticity is a functional, rapid type of plasticity that brings about changes that are usually reversible, while _____ plasticity affects the expression of genotype into phenotype and is not reversible.

9. Cells read genes in two steps: _____, when DNA sequences are copied into RNA, and _____, when information in the RNA produces strings of amino acids.

10. In schizophrenia, the _____ _____ is 50%; this is the rate at which if one twin has schizophrenia, the second will also have it.

DIAGRAM LABELING

Brain Structures

Denote the brain structures on the diagram with the labels listed below the diagram.

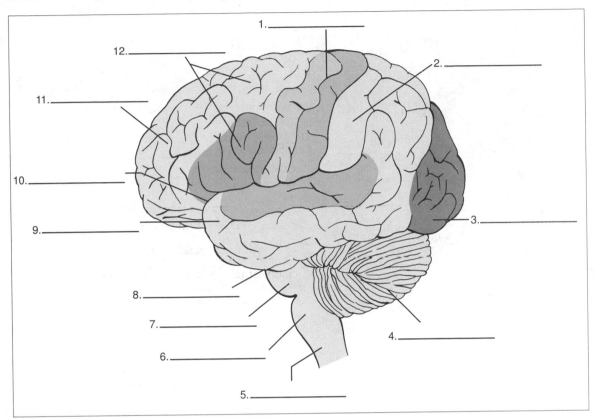

STRUCTURE LABELS:

a. Pons

b. Lateral sulcus

c. Midbrain

d. Central sulcus

e. Parietal lobe

f. Frontal lobe

g. Cerebellum

h. Temporal lobe

i. Medulla oblongata

j. Occipital lobe

k. Gyri

l. Spinal cord

Brain Functions

Denote the brain functions on the diagram with the labels listed below the diagram.

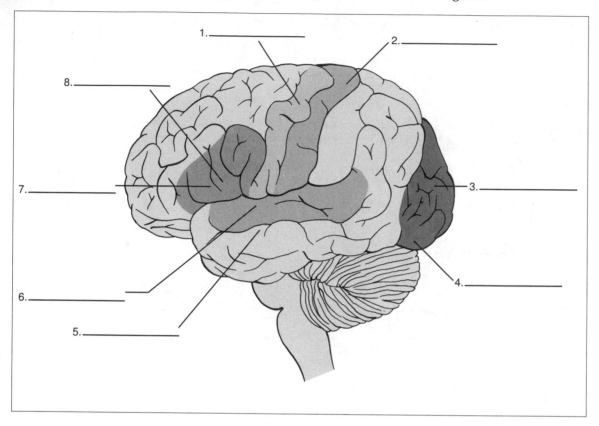

FUNCTION LABELS:

a. Auditory receiving area

b. Written speech

c. Visual interpretation area

d. Visual receiving area

e. Sensory area (pain, touch, etc.)

f. Auditory interpretation area

g. Motor speech

h. Motor cortex

CASE STUDY

Todd is 22 and has just been diagnosed with schizophrenia. He is a twin who was adopted at the age of 6 months. His adoptive father was in the Air Force. Todd's family moved to the Middle East when Todd was 5 years old, and he grew up in a war-torn country until age 10, when his father was transferred back to Washington DC. Todd's twin, Rob, has lived in Milledgeville, Georgia, all his life, and has not evi-denced signs or symptoms of any mental disorders. He is currently an accountant at a local bank. Todd has recently complained of hearing voices and has stayed in his room for about 3 days. He has been sleeping all day and has been up at night. His parents became alarmed and finally brought him to the emergency department when Todd would not come out of his room and would not eat.

1. Explain how Todd and Rob may have genetic tendencies toward schizophrenia, and yet both did not acquire this disease.

2. Which of the neurotransmitters may be most active in creating problems for Todd, and why would it be important to know about this neurotransmitter and its function in the CNS?

3. Discuss at least two brain regions that may be related to Todd's symptoms of hearing voices, withdrawal, not eating and his sleep disturbance.

CRITICAL THINKING AND SELF-EVALUATION EXERCISES

1. Think about your own growth and development. Were there any special occurrences during any of your critical periods of early childhood? Think about how your early experiences might have affected the way you are today as an adult.

2. Have you ever noticed any connections between your immune, psychological, and endocrine systems? Have you ever become sick with a cold or the flu when you were extremely stressed? Think about ways in which your "physical" body might interact with your "mental" or psychological self.

■ NCLEX-Style Exam Questions

1. The most important reason that psychiatric nurses need to know about the brain is that:
   a. it is the organ of the mind and governs all forms of human behavior.
   b. it is the center of all metabolic processes for drugs that are used for psychiatric disorders.
   c. the brain is responsible for the etiology of many mental disorders.
   d. the brain is the central location for transcription of genes related to behavior.

2. In experiments when laboratory mice brains have been depleted of serotonin, the following behaviors were seen:
   a. aggression and hostility.
   b. mating behaviors.
   c. total withdrawal from litter mates.
   d. extraordinary drinking and eating behaviors.

3. One of the most common ways in which neurotransmitters are deactivated within the nervous system at the neuronal level is:
   a. killer cells scavenge the remains of the neurotransmitters.
   b. enzymatic degradation, primarily by monoamine oxidase (MAO).
   c. RNA transferase breaks them down.
   d. the blood-brain barrier ensures that they are deactivated.

4. Mr. Snipes has difficulty with his motor coordination and walks with an unsteady gait. Of the following brain structures, which is most likely affected in Mr. Snipes' brain?
   a. Cerebrum
   b. Medulla oblongata
   c. Hippocampus
   d. Cerebellum

5. Susan cannot remember anything before her accident yesterday. Which brain structure might be injured?
   a. Midbrain
   b. Reticular formation
   c. Basal ganglia
   d. Hippocampus

6. In one study, when kittens were deprived of light and visual stimuli for several weeks prior to and after opening their eyes, and they were not anatomically different from their litter mates, they were rendered blind because:
   a. their visual neurons were never activated for the job of sight through exposure to the visual stimuli needed for them to grow and network.
   b. their visual neurons were never activated because the light deprivation disturbed their circadian rhythm cycles.
   c. their visual neurons were activated, but were not able to perceive light stimuli.
   d. their visual neurons were destroyed because of lack of use.

7. While different brain regions are organizing, they need specific kinds of experiences targeting the region's specific function in order to develop properly. This concept is known as:
   a. functional periods.
   b. neurotransmitter functioning.
   c. critical periods.
   d. Neuroplasticity.

8. Several neuroimaging techniques are available for researchers and practitioners. The value of neuroimaging is that:
   a. it provides data about the actual number of stimuli an individual can take in.
   b. it provides data about the structures of the brain correlated with their activity.

c. it provides information about genetic reproduction of DNA at the time of transcription.

d. It is moderately valuable because it is not
accurate at this point in its development.

9. All but which of the following are currently
used neuroimaging techniques?

a. Computed tomography scans

b. Electrocardiogram tomography

c. Positron-emission tomography

d. Single-photon-emission tomography

10. Jean suffers from seasonal affective disorder
(SAD), in which depression parallels the short-
ening of the days during fall and winter. Which
of the following is most likely affected in Jean?

a. Hippocampus

b. Medulla

c. Circadian rhythm

d. Caudate nucleus and pineal glands

CHAPTER 3

Conceptual Frameworks and Theories

Chapter 3 introduces theories and conceptual frameworks that are useful in psychiatric–mental health nursing. These are worldviews that provide a way of looking at human behavior as well as a systematic way to frame research studies. Several theories have informed the practice of psychiatric nursing. Some examples of such theories include behavior theory, cognitive-behavior theory, biophysiological theory, and sociocultural theories. Research indicates that biologic, psychological, interpersonal, and sociocultural factors play a role in mental illnesses. Researchers have constructed models that go beyond the reductionistic ones of the past to view the individual as a complex organism living, interacting, and transacting with others and negotiating risk and protective factors in his or her ecology. This dynamic view of human beings holds great promise for research and for a more precise assessment and interventions in the future.

LEARNING OBJECTIVES

After completing the exercises in this workbook, and studying the corresponding chapter in the textbook, the student will be able to:

- Describe what is meant by theory and why theories are important to clinical practice.

- Differentiate the psychodynamic, behavioral, cognitive-behavioral, humanistic, sociocultural, biophysiological, and interpersonal theories.

- Give examples of interventions that might be used with a behavioral or cognitive-behavioral approach.

- Describe a conceptual framework that incorporates several theories and its importance to understanding clients in development and context.

KEY TERMS

Applied behavior analysis: A systematic way of examining and analyzing behaviors as they relate to the environment and basing appropriate interventions on this analysis.

Cognitions: Mediating processes that take place between a stimulus and a response.

Concepts: The building blocks of theories.

Conditioning: A basic form of learning by which a subject begins to associate a behavior with a previously unrelated stimulus. There are two kinds of conditioning: operant and respondent.

Countertransference: The feelings and thoughts that a mental health service provider has toward a client that may be related to the provider's own unconscious or repressed emotions, feelings, and experiences.

Defense mechanisms: Unconscious measures that people use to defend their personal stability and protect against anxiety and threat resulting from conflicts between the id, ego, and superego.

Discrimination: The process by which a person learns to distinguish between and respond differently to similar stimuli.

Generalization: The process by which a person learns to associate a conditioned response with similar stimuli.

Hypothesis: An assumptive statement about the relationship between two or more concepts (or variables).

Modeling: The demonstration of desired behavior patterns to a learner.

Operant conditioning: A type of conditioning by which a subject responds to a stimulus to achieve something rewarding or to avoid something aversive.

Punishment: The introduction of an aversive stimulus following a subject's response to decrease the future likelihood of that response.

Reinforcement: The process by which a stimulus, whether pleasant (positive) or aversive (negative), strengthens a new response by its repeated association with that response.

Repressed: Pushed out of consciousness.

Respondent conditioning: The process by which a response and a stimulus become connected.

Shaping: A procedure employed in behavioral therapy when a person lacks a certain behavior in his or her inventory, so that reinforcement of that behavior might take place.

Theory: One person's or a group's beliefs about how something happens or works.

Transference: Feelings and thoughts that a client has toward the nurse, psychiatrist, or other service provider that are rooted in the client's unconscious or repressed emotions and feelings toward people in his or her past (e.g., parents, teachers).

Unconscious: As used by Freud, psychological material that has been repressed.

Utility: The capacity of a theory to generate predictions that are confirmed when relevant empirical data are collected.

Chapter Outline

THEORIES: WHO CARES AND SO WHAT?
THEORIES OF HUMAN BEHAVIOR
Psychoanalytic Perspective
General Principles
Critiques of Psychoanalytic Theory
Behavior Theory
General Principles
   Conditioning
   Reinforcement
   Punishment
   Generalization and Discrimination
   Modeling and Shaping
Applied Behavior Analysis
Cognitive-Behavior Theory
The Humanistic Perspective
The Interpersonal Perspective
The Biophysiological Perspective
The Sociocultural Viewpoint
TOWARD A COMPREHENSIVE, MULTIDISCIPLINARY
   UNDERSTANDING OF PSYCHOPATHOLOGY
The Emergence of Mental Illness
Multidimensionality of Assessment (Assessing Multiple
   Systems)
Family Characteristics (Microsystem)
Community Characteristics (Exosystem)

KEY TOPICS

Why use theories? Definition of theories; uses of theory in practice

Theories of human behavior: Psychodynamic, behavioral, cognitive-behavioral, humanistic, interpersonal, biophysiological, sociocultural

Comprehensive views of psychopathology: Multidisciplinary assessment, including individual, family, and community characteristics

■ Exercises

MATCHING

Match the term in Part A with the statement that applies to the term in Part B:

PART A

a. multidimensional assessment

b. "ABCD" approach in rational-emotive therapy (RET)

c. humanistic perspective in psychiatric mental health

d. Koro

e. an example of psychodynamic principles

f. conditioning

g. operationalization of behavior

h. punishment

i. proximal and distal factors

j. theory

PART B

1. _____ Exploring a particular behavior, and examining the person's beliefs, consequences, and then disputing the maladaptive beliefs.

2. _____ When Jamie lies on the floor and pounds his fists, his parents make him go to his room for a time-out.

3. _____ To change vague words about an event into observable and concrete actions in order to form the basis for behavior change.

4. _____ A worldview of how something happens or works.

5. _____ Holds learning as important as well as other psychological processes, such as creativity, hope, love, self-fulfillment, personal growth, values, and meaning.

6. _____ Jane is unconsciously repressing her feelings of fear about being in a large room.

7. _____ An example of a culture-bound syndrome in which men fear their penis is shrinking.

8. _____ While studying for an exam, a student uses classical music to relax; then, when taking the actual exam, the student's relaxation response "kicks in."

9. _____ Variables that exert the strongest influence on children, and variables that are less influential with children and have less powerful effects.

10. _____ A way of comprehensively addressing the multiple systems that affect the individual, including family and community influences.

COMPLETION

1. One of the major theories that drove the field of psychiatry for decades was _____, and its tenets led some analysts to stop giving medications.

2. You meet a new person who is of interest to you and begin to develop an idea of why that person acts in a particular way. This might be called developing a _____ about that person's behavior.

3. The following statement is an example of a _____: If a person is abused as a small child, then he or she may have lowered self-esteem throughout life.

4. Freud posited that the _____ is completely selfish and wants immediate gratification; the _____ mediates between the id and the external world; and the _____ is your conscience.

5. A patient is exhibiting _____ when he says that you remind him of his sister, who is about your age.

6. Two forms of conditioning are _____ , which happens when a response and a stimulus are connected, and

_____, when individuals respond in order to achieve a certain goal.

7. Providing a pass for a client to go outside into the recreation area because the client finished all her daily chores on the unit would be called _____ reinforcement.

8. In clinical, your instructor speaks with a difficult client in front of you. A behavioral theorist would call this intervention _____.

9. _____ _____ involves helping clients to monitor their beliefs, look for evidence that the beliefs are true, and dispute their maladaptive beliefs in order to change their pattern of distorted thinking.

10. Certain contextual characteristics and events that might block a client's development and adaptation are called _____.

CASE STUDY

Gerri, age 22, grew up in Harlem in New York City. She dropped out of school at age 10 because her parents were both alcoholic and forced her to stay at home to care for her two siblings (ages 2 and 4). Gerri's parents would not allow her to make friends, visit outside her home, or go to any social activities in the neighborhood. Her mother suffered from multiple sclerosis, which caused her to be unable to move easily. The family had no health insurance, and Gerri was frequently asked to go to the local drugstore and steal various medications and remedies. When you first see Gerri, she has been admitted to the inpatient psychiatric unit for treatment of depression. Gerri has not been sleeping or eating well, has lost 10 pounds in the past week, and cries periodically throughout most every day. You have been asked to complete a comprehensive assessment of Gerri's difficulties. Since you are familiar with the Developmental Ecological Model of assessment, you begin to assess Gerri using that approach.

1. On the diagram, fill in the information you have about Gerri that might help you to have a holistic understanding of the life problems that have influenced the development of her depression. Also indicate any missing information that you will obtain later, as you continue to work with Gerri.

Macrosystem

Culture, values, beliefs

Exosystem

Community, geographical environment

Microsystem

Family

Ontogenic

Development, individual

2. As you consider Gerri's life situation and history, briefly outline how each of the following types of theorists would attempt to explain Gerri's depression:

   a. Psychodynamic perspective:

   b. Biophysiological perspective:

   c. Behavioral perspective:

   d. Sociocultural perspective:

CRITICAL THINKING AND SELF-EVALUATION EXERCISES

1. How would you feel about Gerri's life experiences when you met her?

2. What would be your first impression of Gerri, after reading her case study? Can you identify any faulty thoughts or irrational beliefs you might have?

3. Think about your own coping style. Which type of therapy do you think would work best for you (behavioral, psychodynamic, cognitive-behavioral, humanistic, interpersonal, sociocultural), and why?

■ NCLEX-Style Exam Questions

1. In regard to theories, one common mistake that people working in the helping professions make is to:

   a. provide a biological approach to helping with psychiatric disorders by giving several medications at one time.

   b. give medicines along with psychotherapy.

   c. develop an overzealous commitment to one form of therapy, ignoring the benefits that other types of therapies may have for a given individual.

   d. deny access to care by restricting clients to only one form of therapy.

2. Two of the most important reasons that nurses utilize theories in their approach to helping people with psychiatric disorders is that:

   a. theories provide knowledge expansion in the field, and they are a way of incorporating known findings into a framework for understanding clients.

   b. theories help to give a basis for giving certain types of medications, and they also give specific examples of how to help each person.

   c. theories are the basis for reimbursement of health care costs, and they also drive providers' economic motivations for seeking health care.

   d. theories give the nurse examples of how to intervene with patients, and also provide criteria for health care reimbursement.

3. Susan is depressed. A psychoanalytic theorist might say the following about Susan:

   a. Susan may be unconsciously repressing feelings of anger that arise due to her early childhood abuse experiences, and these feelings emerge as depression.

   b. Susan has seen her mother being depressed and has learned that this is one way to receive attention.

   c. When Susan exhibits depressive symptoms, she has always been taken care of by her husband until she is less depressed.

   d. Susan's depression is a result of her poor family upbringing, living in a hostile environment as she was growing up, and frequently seeing violent fighting in her neighborhood.

4. When Bobby, age 3, has a temper tantrum, his parents remove his toys from the playroom for 1 hour. A behavioral theorist would consider this which type of intervention?

   a. Negative reinforcement

   b. Positive reinforcement

   c. Modeling

   d. Punishment

5. When a child's polite behavior (saying please or thank you) happens at home repeatedly, the child is very likely to display that behavior in other circumstances outside the home, given similar conditions. This phenomenon is described as:

   a. generalization.

   b. discrimination.

   c. modeling.

   d. shaping.

6. The "ABCD" approach, used in rational-emotive therapy, includes the following four components:

   a. assessment of behavior; behavior itself; conditioning new behavior; developing consistency.

   b. antecedent behavior; belief; consequence; disputation of maladaptive beliefs.

   c. allowing new behaviors; brainstorming; counseling; deviation assessment.

   d. anonymity; belief; confidentiality; dogma.

7. Interpersonal theorists, such as Harry Stack Sullivan, emphasize which of the following tenets?

   a. The existence of the id, ego, and superego

   b. The importance of conditioning responses in working with people

   c. Interpersonal socialization of humans throughout their developmental stages

   d. Alleviating symptoms by utilizing biological tools, such as medicines

8. The existence of psychiatric syndromes that are seen in non-Western cultures and that are influenced by that culture's social values is called:

   a. medical anthropology.

   b. psychosocial disorder.

   c. social disorders.

   d. culture-bound syndrome.

9. The uniqueness of comprehensive, multidimensional theories for understanding human behavior is that they:

   a. provide more specific answers for the questions around etiology of disorders.

   b. are more confusing than the specific, narrow theories that are often used.

   c. are often misinterpreted as being inclusive of everything that could have an effect on human behavior, and are thus misused.

   d. incorporate several different theoretical viewpoints, and address individual, environmental, and societal characteristics that may influence psychopathology.

10. In the Developmental Ecological Model of understanding behavior, the microsystem (or family) includes which of the following components for assessment?

    a. Family function and structure

    b. Community violence around the family

    c. The family's involvement in church activities

    d. The person's progression through developmental milestones

Therapeutic Relationships and Communication

Chapter 4 is a review of concepts around the therapeutic relationship and communication in psychiatric mental health nursing. Trust, professionalism, mutual respect, caring, and partnership are key elements of a therapeutic nurse–client relationship. Obstacles to effective nurse–client relationships in the psychiatric setting are also explored, including the nurse's judgmental attitudes, excessive probing, and lack of self-awareness. The phases of the therapeutic relationship are the introductory phase, working phase, and termination phase; each phase has a unique set of characteristics and goals. The nurse uses a specific set of listening skills to facilitate communication with clients, while avoiding ineffective listening techniques. Assertiveness and confrontation skills are necessary for communicating effectively and respectfully with psychiatric clients who are in distress. The focus of the therapeutic relationship is on the client's needs, and the nurse should follow strict guidelines for using self-disclosure with clients. Building a therapeutic relationship with the client's family and loved ones is a key component of effective nursing care, while continually examining the self and practice are required to become a skilled, effective, caring professional nurse.

LEARNING OBJECTIVES

After completing the exercises in this workbook, and studying the corresponding chapter in the textbook, the student will be able to:

- List the key ingredients of a therapeutic relationship.

- Identify potential obstacles to the establishment of a therapeutic relationship.

- Describe the three phases of therapeutic relationships.

- Discuss the application of a theoretical model to the components of nurse–client communication.

- Describe effective listening skills to use with clients.

- Contrast effective and ineffective communication techniques with clients.

- Identify techniques for using confrontation and self-assertion with clients.

- Discuss the appropriateness of different levels of self-disclosure with clients.

- Describe the role of the client's family and loved ones in the client's care.

- Analyze case studies that explore specific challenges to establishing therapeutic nurse–client relationships.

KEY TERMS

Aggressiveness: Communication and behavior that are belittling, threatening, moralizing, coercing, or condescending.

Apathy: A sense of detachment and the belief that nothing a person does makes any difference, leading to a lack of concern about the problem or outcome.

Assertiveness: A technique by which a person communicates what he or she thinks, feels, or wants directly and respectfully.

Caring: A core value of nursing that consists of three primary behaviors: 1) giving of self, 2) meeting the client's needs in a timely manner, and 3) providing comfort measures for clients and family members.

Channel: The route or method a communicator chooses to convey his or her message.

Communication: The process of conveying information through a complex variety of verbal and nonverbal behaviors.

Communicator: A person who simultaneously sends and receives messages through words and nonverbal behaviors.

Confrontation: The skill of pointing out, in a caring way, concern about another person's behavior or discrepancies between what the other person says and what he or she does.

Countertransference: The arousal of uncomfortable, sometimes unprofessional feelings within the nurse while he or she is working with clients who present difficult behaviors and dilemmas.

Decoding: The process by which one communicator discerns or interprets what another communicator is saying.

Empathy: Emotional knowing of another person.

Encoding: The process by which a communicator puts into words or behaviors the ideas or feelings that he or she is trying to convey.

Environment: In communication, the personal experiences and cultural background that a communicator brings to an interaction.

External noise: Factors outside a communicator that create distractions.

Feedback: The discernible response that a receiver makes to a sender's message when communicating.

Genuineness: A nursing value that involves being a real person and truly engaged in knowing the client in open, human exchanges.

Listening: Focusing on all behaviors exhibited by a person who is communicating.

Maturity: The ability to integrate aspects of life into a whole and find balance in one's outlook and attitudes toward others.

Noise: Any forces within communicators or in the environment that interfere with effective communication.

Nontherapeutic communication: Interactions in which the nurse uses ineffective responses that result in clients feeling defensive, misunderstood, controlled, minimized, alienated, or discouraged from expressing their thoughts and feelings.

Passive-aggressive communication: Communication that uses indirect aggression through back-stabbing, sabotaging, ignoring, or "forgetting" to do something.

Perception check: A confrontational communication technique that uses a three-step formula to clarify another person's behavior. The three steps are to 1) describe the inconsistent or confusing behavior; 2) offer at least two possible interpretations of that behavior; and 3) ask for feedback.

Physiologic noise: Physical factors within a communicator that detract from effective communication.

Positive reframing: A communication technique in which the mental health care provider specifically states the behavior changes a client should make rather than criticizing the client's negative behavior.

Professional: A person who applies a specific background of knowledge and skills.

Psychological noise: Emotional and cognitive forces within a communicator that interfere with accurately expressing or understanding a message.

Therapeutic communication: A planned process of interaction in which the nurse demonstrates empathy, uses effective communication skills, and responds to the client's thoughts, needs, and concerns.

Transactional analysis: An assertive communication technique by which a person speaks from the adult ego state to others in the adult ego state.

Trust: The risk of sharing oneself with another, knowing that one is opening himself or herself to the possibility of hurt, embarrassment, judgment, and disappointment.

Unconditional positive regard: The ability to give of oneself freely to clients and to see clients as worthy of respect and attention regardless of their behavior, flaws, and setbacks.

Chapter Outline

THERAPEUTIC RELATIONSHIPS
Essential Elements
Trust
Professionalism
Mutual Respect
Caring
Partnership
Obstacles to Establishing a Therapeutic Relationship
Judgmental Attitudes
Excessive Probing
Lack of Self-Awareness
Phases of the Therapeutic Relationship
Introductory Phase
Middle or Working Phase
Termination Phase
THERAPEUTIC COMMUNICATION
Theoretical Framework and Communication Model
Listening
Assertiveness
Confrontation and Limit-Setting
Self-Disclosure
Therapeutic Communication in Special Situations
Clients with Anxiety
Clients with Psychoses
Families

KEY TOPICS

Therapeutic relationship: Essential elements (trust, professionalism, mutual respect, caring, partnership); obstacles to establishing (judgmental attitudes, excessive probing, lack of self-awareness); phases (introductory, middle, and termination)

Therapeutic communication: Theoretical framework and communication model

Therapeutic communication techniques: Listening, assertiveness, confrontation and setting limits; self-disclosure

Therapeutic communication with special populations: Clients with anxiety, psychoses; families

■ Exercises

MATCHING

Match the therapeutic technique in Part A with the example in Part B.

PART A

a. giving broad openings

b. paraphrasing

c. offering a general lead

d. reflecting feelings

e. focusing

f. voicing doubt

g. clarifying

h. placing events into a time sequence

i. giving information

j. encouraging formation of a plan

k. testing discrepancies

PART B

1. _____ "Yes, I see." "Uh-huh."

2. _____ "I'm not sure what you mean by 'going under.'"

3. _____ "What do you think your options are to deal with this problem?" "Let's list some possibilities for how you can get to the sessions."

4. _____ "It sounds as if you are growing tired of always trying to placate your husband."

5. _____ "Are you certain that your boss would never accept your reason for doing it that way?" "Really?"

6. _____ "How did this behavior first begin?" "What happened after that?"

7. _____ "What you are saying is that your children don't really follow your directions or obey instructions when you speak to them?"

8. _____ "Can you specify exactly what it is about your school that bothers you?"

9. _____ "You stated that you wanted to come each week, but I notice that you usually miss every other week's appointment."

10. _____ "Can you describe how your week has gone here on the unit?"

11. _____ "It takes 1 to 2 weeks for your medication to take effect."

SHORT ANSWER

For each nontherapeutic communication technique listed below, provide the purpose and an example for each.

1. Social responding

   a. Purpose: _____

   b. Example: _____

2. Closed-ended questions

   a. Purpose: _____

   b. Example: _____

3. Changing the subject

   a. Purpose: _____

   b. Example: _____

4. Belittling

   a. Purpose: _____

   b. Example: _____

5. Making stereotyped comments

   a. Purpose: _____

   b. Example: _____

6. False reassurance

   a. Purpose: _____

   b. Example: _____

7. Moralizing

   a. Purpose: _____

   b. Example: _____

8. Interpreting

   a. Purpose: _____

   b. Example: _____

9. Advising

   a. Purpose: _____

   b. Example: _____

10. Challenging

   a. Purpose: _____

   b. Example: _____

11. Defending

   a. Purpose: _____

   b. Example: _____

CORRECT THE FALSE STATEMENTS

1. Despite the incredible developments in technology that hold promise for treatment of psychiatric disorders, the primary medium through which all psychiatric care is provided is still the administration of appropriate biological therapies, such as medications.

2. Anonymity is a component of trust, and includes the right for clients to conceal that they are receiving treatment for a mental health problem.

3. Trust consists of three primary behaviors: giving of the self, meeting the client's needs in a timely manner, and providing comfort measures for clients and their families.

4. Sympathy involves listening carefully, being in tune with what clients are saying, and having insight into the meaning of their thoughts, feelings, and behaviors.

5. The nurse exhibits lack of self-awareness when she states, "I think Joan should just pull herself up by her bootstraps; she isn't even trying to help herself."

CASE STUDY

Jamie is a 24-year-old schoolteacher who is admitted to the psychiatric unit by a police officer. After "binge drinking" last night, which resulted in her passing out, she awoke with a severe anxiety attack because she did not know where she was. She has experienced mild "panic attacks" (as she describes them) in the past, but this one is worse than any before. It appeared to Jamie that perhaps she had

been raped, which brought back memories of an experience of abuse at the age of 12. She was aching all over, was undressed, and began to hear a radio playing in her head. She dialed 911 on a phone in the room and was picked up by a police officer, who brought her to the emergency department. She was screened for rape in the ED, but there was no evidence of rape.

When she arrives on your unit, Jamie is disheveled and states very anxiously that the radio noise in her head "just won't stop!" She is shaking, is sweating mildly, and complains of a racing heartbeat with difficulty breathing. When you introduce yourself to Jamie, she seems to ignore you, or seems not to even hear you speaking.

1. What do you think might be potential obstacles for a nurse who is trying to establish a therapeutic relationship with Jamie?

2. What attitudes from the nurse's cultural and personal background might potentially interfere with his or her ability to convey an accepting, nonjudgmental approach to Jamie?

3. What types of actions might be most appropriate in the nurse's first interview with Jamie that would help to establish rapport, define the parameters of the relationship, and reduce Jamie's anxiety?

4. Discuss the phase of the therapeutic relationship the nurse and Jamie are in on admission, including the focus of this phase, and helpful nursing interventions that are appropriate to this phase of the therapeutic relationship.

Nursing Process Exercise

Prepare a nursing care plan that would be aimed toward meeting goals of the initial phase of your therapeutic relationship with Jamie. Prior to developing a working nursing diagnosis, you complete a comprehensive assessment of Jamie. Highlight or underline the data provided in the scenario description above that you will use to assess Jamie. Note any additional information that you will need to gather at a later date. With the data you have from the scenario above, work on a nursing care plan for Jamie for the first 8 hours of her admission. Use the nursing diagnosis worksheet to complete the sections, as follows:

NURSING PROCESS WORKSHEET[1]

Health Problem (Title)	**Client Goal***
Related to ↓	
Etiology (Related Factors)	**Nursing Interventions***
Evidenced by ↓	
Signs and Symptoms (Defining Characteristics)	**Evaluative Statement**

[1]Refer to textbook, Chapter 6, for more information about Care Planning.

*More than one client goal may be appropriate. For this exercise, choose one client goal that demonstrates a direct resolution of the client problem identified in the nursing diagnosis.

**Be sure you are able to list the scientific rationale for each nursing intervention you order.

Nursing Diagnosis

Under "Health Problem" describe Jamie's most immediate health problem upon admission. Use your textbook as a reference for diagnoses that may be specific to Jamie's presenting problem. Then, fill in the blank under "Etiology," listing relevant factors that may be related to Jamie's problem. The related factors that you list here identify Jamie's specific circumstance and will direct the selection of nursing interventions. Under "Signs & Symptoms," list those that were mentioned in the scenario above. These are subjective and objective data that must be present in order to substantiate using the diagnosis you used.

Planning

For the "Client Goal," often referred to as the outcome, state one goal for Jamie that would be most relevant for the first 8 hours of care. Remember: goal statements must be realistic, measurable, and expected as an outcome of nursing care, and must have a realistic timeline. Goals should be stated in behavioral terms; the verb used in the statement must represent a behavior of Jamie that can be observed.

Intervention

"Nursing Interventions" are activities that the nurse will complete to help Jamie achieve the goal you identified above. There are many potential nursing interventions that may be appropriate for a given client goal. Optimally, you should list several interventions that will assist Jamie to move toward her goal.

Evaluative Statement

The "Evaluative Statement," or evaluation section, in the nursing care plan is very important because it documents Jamie's progress toward meeting her goal. Each time Jamie completes a behavior that indicates her progress, it should be noted in the evaluation portion of the care plan. Also, if there are interventions that are not helpful for Jamie, this should also be noted. Remember, the purpose of your care plan is to guide your nursing interventions in a meaningful manner, as well as to assist other caregivers to understand and to be able to implement the plan of care for your client when you are not there.

■ NCLEX-Style Exam Questions

1. Which theorist was most widely known for her belief that the cornerstone of all nursing care is the therapeutic relationship?

   a. Jean Watson
   b. Hildegard Peplau
   c. Florence Nightingale
   d. Clara Barton

2. A psychiatric nurse tells her client that she will return in 15 minutes to talk with him. She goes to a meeting that runs overtime and returns in an hour, apologizing for being late. This behavior may have an impact between the nurse and her client in the area of:

   a. establishing confidentiality
   b. establishing boundaries on the therapeutic relationship.
   c. getting through the working phase of the relationship.
   d. establishing trust in the introductory phase of the relationship.

3. One of the most common reasons that clients are often concerned about confidentiality of their treatment for a mental health problem is that:

   a. they lack health care coverage for the treatment.
   b. they are worried about the opinions of people who know them outside the hospital, due to shame produced by societal views of mental illness.
   c. they do not understand that most people will not know what a mental health problem is.
   d. they are concerned about receiving their next paycheck when they return to work.

4. Psychiatric nurses often feel a heightened sense of respect for clients when they realize how clients have struggled with extraordinary events and disabling symptoms. This is an example of:

   a. empathic response to therapy.
   b. professionalism, maturity, and mutual respect.
   c. setting boundaries between the client and society.
   d. caregiver sympathy.

5. Caring, one of the core values of nursing, consists of all but which of the following primary behaviors?

   a. Giving of the self
   b. Setting boundaries within the relationship
   c. Meeting the client's needs in a timely manner

d. Providing comfort measures to clients and their families

6. Empathy involves all but which of the following?

   a. Careful listening

   b. Being in touch with what clients are saying

   c. Having insight into the meaning of clients' thoughts, feelings, and behaviors

   d. Feeling the same emotions that the client is feeling at a given time

7. Jane, a nursing student, is working with Todd, an alcoholic. Although Jane has an aversive feeling toward people who abuse alcohol, she feels that Todd is worthy of respect and attention regardless of her own personal feelings. This is an example of:

   a. unconditional positive regard.

   b. countertransference.

   c. partnership.

   d. genuineness.

8. All except which of the following statements would indicate that the nurse has a judgmental attitude?

   a. "People who are mentally ill have basically weak characters."

   b. "I think Susan is exaggerating her feelings so she can leave work early."

   c. "Mental illnesses are, for the most part, all in your head and could be solved more easily if people were forced to continue with their daily activities, instead of listening to their complaints."

   d. "Cindy has struggled with her life circumstance of living with a man who beats her, and she is trying very hard to make the changes necessary to help herself."

9. Carrie, a nursing student, is caring for a man who has been arrested for child abuse. She is very curious about what he must have done to get into so much trouble, so she asks him to tell her about the various activities that got him arrested. This is an example of:

   a. lack of awareness.

   b. genuineness and caring.

   c. gathering assessment data.

   d. excessive probing.

10. All except which of the following are goals of the working phase of the therapeutic relationship?

    a. Identify past behaviors that have been ineffective for coping with the focal problem

    b. Reduce the client's anxieties

    c. Increase hopefulness for the future

    d. Develop a plan of action, practice it, and evaluate its effectiveness

CHAPTER 5

Culture

This chapter discusses culture, which is a main ingredient of personality. The more stress a person experiences, the greater is the manifestation of his or her culturally based perceptions, beliefs, and behaviors. Self-knowledge facilitates personal comfort and understanding of others when caring for culturally diverse clients in a variety of psychiatric–mental health settings. To provide effective, individualized mental health services, nurses must view consumers with a cultural lens that includes the context of their cultural group and their individual experiences from being a part of that group. Although diverse cultural groups may have various health care responses to mental illness, culturally competent care is maximized by the nurse's open, honest, and accepting attitude. Nurses' self-knowledge, viewing position, and preparation as culturally competent providers greatly affect the care of diverse clients.

LEARNING OBJECTIVES

After completing the exercises in this workbook, and studying the corresponding chapter in the textbook, the student will be able to:

- Describe the importance of culture to human behavior and its effect on the provision of effective mental health services.

- Explain how demographic changes in North America are contributing to the importance of cultural awareness.

- Describe the elements of a culturally congruent service system.

- Identify disparities in mental health for clients from minority cultures.

- Explore possible barriers that have led to mental health disparities for clients from minority cultures.

- Discuss biologic variations and various social, psychological, and spiritual perspectives within ethnic groups and across cultures.

- Identify the important aspects of transcultural assessment.

- Describe skills essential to the implementation of culturally competent care.

- Explain nurses' unique position in providing culturally competent care.

- Assess one's own heritage, reference group, and personal and cultural biases.

KEY TERMS

Assimilation: The prevailing expectation during most of the 20th century for immigrants and minority groups in the United States to become like the majority (white) culture.

Cultural competence: The skills, both academic and interpersonal, that allow persons to understand and appreciate cultural differences and similarities within, between, and among groups.

Culture: The integration of human behavior (including thoughts, communications, actions, customs, beliefs, values, and institutions) of a racial, ethnic, religious, or social group.

Culture-bound: A term used to describe a person whose understanding of other cultures is limited because he or she refuses to go beyond the parameters of his or her personal culture.

Culture care theory: A theory developed by Dr. Madeleine Leininger that emphasizes learning principles related to culture care, cultural assessments, the universality of culture care diversity, and the importance of fit between the client's health care values and services provided.

Discrimination: Differential treatment based on race, class, gender, or other variables rather than on individual merit.

Ethnocentrism: The belief that one's own cultural practices and values are inherently correct or superior to those of others.

Flexibility: The ability to embrace change by modifying expectations, readjusting old operating norms and stereotypes, and trying new behavior.

Prejudice: Negative preconceived opinions about other people or groups based on hearsay, perception, or emotion.

Stereotyping: Believing that one member of a cultural group will display certain behaviors or hold certain attitudes (usually negative) simply because he or she is a member of that cultural group.

Stigmatization: The attribution of negative characteristics or identity to one person or group, causing the person or group to feel rejected, alienated, and ostracized from society.

Chapter Outline

CULTURE
Changing Demographics and Cultural Awareness
Assimilation
Implications for Health Care
Culturally Competent Health Care
Cultural Congruence
Culture Care Theory
DISPARITIES IN MENTAL HEALTH AND BARRIERS TO EFFECTIVE TREATMENT
Variability and Vulnerability
Accessibility
Racial Bias
Religious and Spiritual Influences
SOCIOCULTURAL VARIATIONS IN RESPONSE TO MENTAL HEALTH CARE
African Americans
Native Americans
Hispanic and Latino Clients
Asian and Pacific Islanders
CULTURALLY COMPETENT AND CONGRUENT NURSING CARE
Essential Skills
Phases of Transcultural Nursing Knowledge
Transcultural Assessment
Building Cultural Awareness
Cultural Self-Awareness

KEY TOPICS

Culture: Changing demographics and cultural awareness; disparities in mental health care and barriers to effective treatment

Sociocultural variations in response to mental health care: How different cultures respond to treatment and perceive mental disorders: African Americans, Native Americans, Hispanic and Latino clients, and Asian and Pacific Islanders

Culturally competent and congruent nursing care: Essential skills; transcultural nursing knowledge and assessment; how to build cultural awareness and self-awareness

■ Exercises

MATCHING

Match the term in Part A with the statement that applies to the term in Part B.

PART A

a. culture
b. culture-bound
c. assimilation
d. cultural competence
e. discrimination
f. prejudice
g. stigmatization
h. ethnocentrism
i. stereotyping
j. cultural congruence

PART B

1. _____ Being limited by the boundaries and parameters of one's own culture

2. _____ Differential treatment based on race, class, gender, or other variables rather than on individual merit

3. _____ When people in a system (such as health care) receive an overall message of personal and cultural validation

4. _____ Integration of human behaviors of a racial, ethnic, religious, or social group

5. _____ To attribute negative characteristics to one person/group, causing them to feel rejected, alienated, and ostracized from society

6. _____ Believing that one member of a cultural group will display certain behaviors simply because he/she is a member of that group

7. _____ Belief that one's own culture is correct or superior to any others

8. _____ The expectation that immigrants and minorities will become like the dominant (white) culture

9. _____ Preconceived, negative opinions about other people/groups based on hearsay, perception, or emotion

10. _____ Skills that allow a person to understand and appreciate cultural differences and similarities between and within groups

Match the selected descriptors of the particular group with its cultural heritage.

1. _____ African American

2. _____ Native American

3. _____ Hispanic and Latino clients

4. _____ Asian and Pacific Islanders

a. Most likely to use formal mental health services primarily during crisis; Catholic church is important, as are prayers, herbs, and strong influence of hot/cold or good/evil imbalances in promoting a sense of well-being

b. Wide and varied attitudes and beliefs, largely dependent on the individual client; may face racial bias that causes providers to misdiagnose (and mistreat) their disorders

c. Over 30 different ethnic subgroups; tend to endure stress for long periods prior to seeking mental health services; therefore many will have more severe disturbances when they enter the health care system; some groups suffer disproportionately from post-traumatic stress disorder

d. Many different tribes; use traditional herbs and healing practices; most likely to comply with a treatment approach that allows them to preserve their familiar practices

SHORT ANSWER

There are four critical skills that nurses must acquire to provide culturally competent care. For each of the critical skills listed below, provide a brief description of its meaning and an example of how to incorporate each skill into your nursing practice.

1. Cross-cultural understanding: _____

_____

_____

_____

2. Intercultural communication: _____

_____

_____

_____

_____

3. Facilitation skills: _____

_____

_____

_____

_____

4. Flexibility: _____

_____

_____

_____

_____

SELF-AWARENESS EXERCISE

Consider your own upbringing and the culture in which you grew up. What is your awareness of cultural norms, beliefs, and values in your own family? Answer each of the following questions.

• What ethnic group, socioeconomic class, and community do I belong to or feel a part of?
• To what extent do I recognize and understand my own racial or ethnic background?
• What are the values of my ethnic group(s)? What do we generally believe about mental health and mental illness?
• What are my earliest images of race and color?
• What are my attitudes toward people who are different from me in appearance and behavior?
• What have been my personal experiences with others' ethnic or racial cultures?
• What do I know about people from ethnic groups that are different from my own?
• Many nurses and clients are descendants of several racial or ethnic cultures. How do different racial or ethnic cultures come together in my own background?

■ NCLEX-Style Exam Questions

1. According to the U.S. Census Bureau, the following is true regarding changing demographics in America:
   a. There are fewer immigrants coming into the U.S. than ever before in American history.
   b. Over the next 50 years, the number of Hispanics is projected to more than double in America.
   c. Over the next 20 years, the minority population in America will be Caucasian.
   d. The number of Native Americans will more than double in the next 10 years.

2. The statement, "Your 2-year-old daughter must be taught to speak English or she will not be able to succeed in school" is an example of:
   a. stereotyping.
   b. assimilation.
   c. prejudice.
   d. stigmatization.

3. All except which of the following problems stems from ethnocentric attitudes?
   a. Prejudice
   b. Cultural congruence
   c. Stereotyping
   d. Stigmatization

4. Susan makes certain that her client Maria, who is Hispanic, is able to attend Mass each Sunday morning in the hospital chapel. Maria had asked Susan to help her get to Mass. This is an example of:
   a. culturally competent health care.
   b. differential treatment based on religious beliefs.
   c. favoritism among clients on the unit in which Susan works.
   d. ethnocentrism, because Susan is also Catholic.

5. In the U.S. Department of Health and Human Services' published recommendations for providing culturally congruent health care services, all but which of the following are included?

   a. Reach consensus regarding terminology
   b. Distinguish between cultural identification and the culture of poverty
   c. Develop skills based on values to develop culturally congruent services
   d. Develop service subunits that are specific to each cultural group served

6. Racial bias is evident in mental health care treatment, as reflected by which of the following?
   a. Nonwhite clients are institutionalized much more frequently than are whites.
   b. White clients are given access to better facilities within most mental health treatment centers.
   c. It is increasingly difficult to receive reimbursement for mental health services.
   d. Most nonwhite clients are grossly undermedicated when treated in inpatient facilities.

7. All except which of the following are considered traditional healers?
   a. Curandera
   b. Sezuadora
   c. Sobadoras
   d. Brujas

8. Cross-cultural understanding is evidenced by which of the following?
   a. Marsha, a new nurse, has a client who speaks Spanish; she has asked her Hispanic colleague to tell her about the culture, ideas for care, and how cultural beliefs might influence her client's response to health care interventions.
   b. Harriet, an experienced nurse, states during a nursing report meeting, "I just don't feel it is appropriate to allow Hector to attend Mass when everyone else has to stay here."
   c. Sharon has independently formed a prayer group on the unit for all clients who are Catholic.
   d. Jim has begun a client teaching group entitled, "Understanding Your Medications."

9. Flexibility is a critical skill for nurses in providing culturally competent care. In this context, flexibility means:
   a. the nurse can move from one client to another and understand that particular client's cultural values and beliefs immediately.

b. the nurse can change his or her expectations, norms, and stereotypes and try out new behaviors.

c. the nurse can educate her client from any cultural group in a way that conforms to that client's cultural beliefs.

d. the nurse knows major concepts about each cultural group and how their cultural beliefs affect attitudes toward mental health care.

10. Erik Erikson defined the final stage of human development as:

a. coming to terms with one's own cultural identity.

b. trust vs. mistrust.

c. coming to terms with one's own mortality.

d. ego integration vs. despair.

CHAPTER 6

The Nursing Process in Psychiatric–Mental Healthcare

This chapter reviews and discusses the nursing process in relationship to psychiatric nursing care. Nursing assessment involves gathering client data and exploring the needs, problems, and adaptive resources of the individual. In psychiatric nursing particularly, the nurse's communication and relationship skills are essential in conducting an assessment interview. Analysis of client assessment data results in determination of important, clearly written, definitive nursing diagnoses. The nursing diagnosis is a statement of a client's response pattern to a health disruption and guides the planning and intervention phases of the nursing process. The DSM-IV is a multi-axial classification system that fosters a holistic approach to the client; it includes specific behavioral criteria for each psychiatric diagnosis. The current NANDA taxonomy contains nursing diagnoses useful for psychiatric nursing. Nursing care plans define the goals or outcomes of care and the methods to achieve them. Intervention requires nurses to combine data from plans of care with information from what is occurring at the moment, prioritize client needs, and then match this information with an appropriate therapeutic strategy. In evaluation, the final phase of the nursing process, nurses determine the effectiveness of an intervention or the attainment of a preset goal.

LEARNING OBJECTIVES

After completing the exercises in this workbook, and studying the corresponding chapter in the textbook, the student will be able to:

- Apply the nursing process to the practice of psychiatric–mental health nursing.

- Explain the components of a psychosocial assessment.

- Describe the importance of the interview in the assessment process.

- Explain a focused assessment approach by which to structure a psychosocial assessment.

- List several nursing diagnoses that may apply to the care of clients with psychiatric disorders.

- Explain the use of the multi-axial system of psychiatric diagnoses of the Diagnostic and Statistical

Manual of Mental Disorders, fourth edition (DSM-IV-TR).

- Discuss how to organize and use psychosocial assessment data in formulating nursing care plans.

- Explain the use of standardized nursing care plans and clinical pathways in mental health care.

- Describe the critical thinking process that shapes moment-to-moment interventions with clients.

- Explain the relationship of evaluation to the other phases of the nursing process.

KEY TERMS

Assessment: Gathering, classifying, categorizing, analyzing, and documenting information about a client's health status.

Behavioral statement: A statement in a nursing plan of care in which the verb represents an observable behavior.

Diagnostic and Statistical Manual of Mental Disorders (DSM): A criteria-based psychiatric diagnostic system that specifies the type, intensity, duration, and effect of the various behaviors and symptoms required for the diagnosis.

Mental status examination: A tool for assessing objective and observational data that yields information about the client's appearance, level of consciousness, motor status and behavior, affect and mood, attitude, intellectual functioning, speech, cognitive status (including attention and concentration), judgment, abstraction, content of thought, and insight.

Nursing diagnosis: A clinical judgment about individual, family, or community responses to actual or potential health problems or life processes; it is the product of the analysis of data collected during the assessment step of the nursing process.

Nursing process: A problem-solving method of five steps (assessment, nursing diagnosis, planning, intervention, and evaluation) that nurses systematically apply to the care of clients.

Objective data: Phenomena that a person other than the client observes to be present.

Psychosocial assessment: The assessment of psychological, sociological, developmental, spiritual, and cultural data commonly derived from interviews with a client.

Subjective data: Data that the nurse gathers by interviewing the client.

Taxonomy: A classification system that uses a hierarchical structure.

Variance: Anything that alters the client's progress through a normal critical pathway; examples include an unexpected complication or an unusual occurrence in the care delivery system.

Chapter Outline

STEPS OF THE NURSING PROCESS
Assessment
Components of the Psychosocial Assessment
   Interview
   Health History
   Mental Status Examination
Nursing Diagnosis
The NANDA Taxonomy
Choosing and Formulating the Nursing Diagnosis
Nursing Diagnosis and Psychiatric Diagnosis
Planning
Identifying Outcomes
Selecting Interventions
   Standardized Care Plans
   Clinical or Critical Pathways
Implementation
Intervention Strategies for Beginning Practitioners
Supervision
Evaluation

KEY TOPICS

Steps of the nursing process: Assessment, nursing diagnosis, planning, implementation, evaluation

Assessment: Includes psychosocial assessment (interview, health history, and mental status examination)

Diagnosis: Nursing diagnosis uses the NANDA taxonomy; psychiatric diagnosis uses the DSM-IV-TR taxonomy

Planning: Includes identifying outcomes, and selecting interventions (using individualized and/or standardized care plans, and critical/clinical pathways)

Implementation: Intervention strategies and clinical supervision in psychiatric mental health

Evaluation: Includes evaluating client outcomes against goals that have been set.

■ Exercises

MATCHING

Match the category of the Mental Status Examination with its definition in Part A and questions that could be used to elicit that information in Part B.

MENTAL STATUS EXAM CATEGORIES

a. orientation

b. sensorium

c. appearance and behavior

d. speech and communication

e. mood

f. affect

g. thinking

h. perception

i. memory

j. judgment

k. insight

Part A: Definitions

Place the letter in the appropriate definition blank, using each only once.

1. _____ Describes a client's wakefulness or consciousness

2. _____ Level of awareness and orientation

3. _____ Observable characteristics of a person

4. _____ The subjective way a client explains feelings

5. _____ The mind's ability to recall earlier events

6. _____ Way a person experiences his or her environment; equivalent to a sense of reality; derived from the senses of vision, hearing, touch, smell, and taste

7. _____ A person's display of emotion or feelings

8. _____ A person's ability to form valid conclusions and behave in a socially appropriate manner

9. _____ The process or way of thinking or analysis of the world; way of connecting or associating thoughts; overall organization of thoughts

10. _____ Awareness of one's own responsibilities; the ability to objectively analyze the problem

11. _____ How the client is communicating; including rate, volume, modulation, and flow

Part B: Ways to Elicit Information

Place the letter in the appropriate blank; you may use the same letter twice.

1. _____ Evaluate the client's communication with you, not so much what he is saying.

2. _____ Can you see or hear things that other people do not know are there?

3. _____ What would you do if a policeman stopped you for speeding?

4. _____ What is the time? Date? Where are you?

5. _____ What has your mood been like lately?

6. _____ What did you do yesterday? Do you remember my name?

7. _____ Do you have trouble concentrating or focusing your thoughts?

8. _____ Observe what the client is wearing, unusual physical characteristics, activity.

9. _____ Have you been more or less emotional than usual lately?

10. _____ What do you think is the real problem that resulted in you being here?

11. _____ Are there thoughts you cannot get out of your mind? Do you have trouble keeping up with your thoughts or understanding them?

STEPS OF NURSING PROCESS EXERCISE

For each of the five steps of the nursing process, use the chart to provide a description of the step in your own words, and give an example of each as you would find it in a client's chart.

Step of Nursing Process	Description of Step	Example of Step
ASSESSMENT		
DIAGNOSIS		
PLANNING		
IMPLEMENTATION		
EVALUATION		

CORRECT THE NURSING DIAGNOSIS STATEMENTS

For each of the incorrect nursing diagnoses in the chart, change it to a correct diagnosis by inserting the appropriate statements. An example is provided for the first diagnosis.

Incorrect	Correct
Depression related to death of best friend.	*Dysfunctional grieving related to lack of support secondary to death of best friend, as evidenced by the statement, "I now have nowhere to go and no one to talk to."*
Risk for Self-Mutilation related to being alone	
Disturbed sleep Pattern related to discomfort on hospital bed.	
Ineffective Family Coping related to lack of communication betweeen client and her parents.	

■ NCLEX-Style Exam Questions

1. In planning care for clients, the RN uses the nursing process, which is based upon:
   a. a variety of theoretical approaches.
   b. the psychosocial assessment of the client.
   c. the scientific method.
   d. a comprehensive physical and psychological assessment of the client.

2. The five steps of the nursing process, in order, are:
   a. assessment, diagnosis, planning, implementation, and evaluation.
   b. organize data, identify problems, nursing care plan, execution of the plan, and evaluation of outcomes.
   c. planning, diagnosis, implementation, evaluation, and outcome identification.
   d. outcome identification, assessment, diagnosis, implementation, and evaluation.

3. The single most important source of information in the nurse's psychosocial assessment of the client is:
   a. the client's chart, containing past history.
   b. the client's understanding of his/her difficulties.
   c. the family's knowledge about the client and his/her behaviors.
   d. initial and ongoing interviews with the client and family.

4. The following statement written by the RN: "The client appears disheveled and smells of alcohol" would appear under which of the following?

    a. Mental status examination

    b. Observations

    c. Assessment of client's potential health problems

    d. History

5. Nursing diagnosis is defined by NANDA as:

    a. "the identification of core areas of concern for the client."

    b. "a clinical judgment about the client's, family's, or community's potential need for services."

    c. "a clinical judgment about individual, family, or community responses to actual or potential health problems/life processes."

    d. "a judgment about psychosocial and physical areas for nursing interventions."

6. Which of the following is an accurate nursing diagnostic statement, according to NANDA?

    a. Ineffective Individual Coping related to inability to trust others, evidenced by the client remaining in room during meals and stating, "I don't like to be with other people."

    b. Depression related to ineffective coping, evidenced by feelings of sadness and suicidal ideation

    c. Hyperactivity related to manic episode, evidenced by running up and down the hallways with few clothes on

    d. Potential for Abuse of Others related to recent fist fight, evidenced by client's statement, "If I can't get what I want, I'll just fight for my rights!"

7. The stage of Planning involves which of the following?

    a. Selecting appropriate interventions and evaluating the client's response

    b. Using evidence-based interventions and evaluative methods to ascertain the client's needs

    c. Assessing the client's response to prior interventions

    d. Outcome identification and intervention selection

8. All except which of the following are considered appropriate nursing interventions for the RN practicing at a basic (BSN) level?

    a. Milieu therapy

    b. Consultation

    c. Health teaching

    d. Case management

9. For beginning practitioners, all except which of the following would be appropriate intervention strategies?

    a. Problem-solving approach

    b. Crisis intervention

    c. Stress management

    d. Defense mechanism identification

10. The best data for evaluating the client's response to nursing interventions comes from:

    a. the client's family's reports of how the client is changing in a positive fashion.

    b. the observation and documentation of client behaviors.

    c. suggestions of the nursing care team about which interventions are working.

    d. group meetings between the client and the care team.

CHAPTER 7

Legal and Ethical Aspects of Psychiatric–Mental Health Nursing

This chapter introduces and discusses concepts related to legal and ethical issues in psychiatric mental health. A failure to meet the standard of care that results in an injury to a client or consumer makes the nurse liable for nursing negligence or malpractice. To provide legally acceptable nursing care in psychiatric–mental health settings, nurses must be informed about a variety of legal issues, including client rights, and nurses must take responsibility, along with other health team members, to see that client rights are protected. Nurses have the responsibility to understand ethical theories and to follow ethical principles in providing care to the psychiatric client. Psychiatric–mental health nurses put ethics into practice every day when they demonstrate respect within the therapeutic relationship and when they protect and build the client's dignity. Autonomy, beneficence, paternalism, veracity, fidelity, and justice are ethical principles used by psychiatric nurses in ethical decision-making. Boundaries are essential in therapeutic relationships, and nurses must evaluate and maintain the boundaries in the nurse–client relationship.

LEARNING OBJECTIVES

After completing the exercises in this workbook, and studying the corresponding chapter in the textbook, the student will be able to:

- Identify basic legal issues related to psychiatric–mental health nursing care.

- Explain the role of nurse practice acts in terms of legal concerns.

- Discuss issues related to malpractice and measures that health care professionals can take to protect themselves from litigation.

- Discuss the basic rights of people with mental illness.

- Describe different types of commitments and states of competency.

- Describe standard of care as a concept in practice.

- Discuss ethics as they apply to psychiatric–mental health nursing practice.

- Explain the American Nurses Association's code for nurses.

- Analyze the ethical principles of autonomy, beneficence, paternalism, veracity, and fidelity in relation to the care of the client with a psychiatric disorder.

- Describe the role of ethics in community practice settings.

- Discuss situations in which there is a conflict between two or more ethical principles.

KEY TERMS

Autonomy: The right to make decisions for oneself.

Battery: Touching another person without his or her permission.

Beneficence: The principle of doing good, not harm.

Emergency admission: Admission to a psychiatric hospital that occurs when a client acts in a way that indicates that he or she is mentally ill and, as a consequence of the particular illness, is likely to harm self or others. State statutes define the exact procedure for the initial evaluation and the possible length of detainment.

Ethical dilemma: A situation in which there are conflicting moral claims or in which two ethical principles conflict.

Ethics: Principles that serve as a code of conduct about right and wrong behavior to guide the actions of individuals.

Fidelity: Faithfulness to duties, obligations, and promises.

Informed consent: Consent that a recipient of health care gives to treating providers that enables the recipient to understand a proposed treatment, including its administration, prognosis after treatment, side effects, risks, possible consequences of refusal, and other alternatives.

Involuntary admission: Admission to a psychiatric hospital that occurs when a person with mental illness who refuses psychiatric hospitalization or treatment poses a danger to self or others and cannot safely be cared for in a less restrictive setting.

Malpractice: A tort action that a consumer plaintiff brings against a defendant professional from whom the plaintiff believes that he or she has received injury during the course of the professional–consumer relationship; professional negligence.

Paternalism: An ethical principle by which the intent is to do good; however, the professional determines what is considered "good" and may override a client's wishes and self-determination.

Reasonable person test: A legal concept that refers to how a reasonable and prudent health care professional is expected to perform with regard to his or her professional role in a practice situation.

Respondeat superior: A Latin term meaning that acts of employees are attributable to their employer, whom the court also will find responsible for damages to injured third parties.

Substituted consent: Authorization that another person gives on behalf of a client who needs a procedure or treatment but cannot provide consent for it independently.

Veracity: A systematic display of honesty and truthfulness in speech.

Voluntary admissions: An admission to a psychiatric hospital that occurs (1) through a client's direct request by coming to the hospital or (2) following evaluation of a client who is determined dangerous to self or others or unable to adequately meet his or her own needs in the community, but is willing to submit to treatment and is competent to do so.

Chapter Outline

LEGAL ISSUES IN PSYCHIATRIC–MENTAL HEALTH NURSING CARE
Nurse Practice Acts and the Expanding Role of Nursing
Malpractice
Obtaining Legal Counsel
Basic Rights of Clients Receiving Psychiatric Nursing Care
Informed Consent
   Special Considerations in Psychiatric Settings
   Substituted Consent
Confidentiality
   Responsible Record Keeping
   Privileged Communication
Evolving Legal Rights
Right to Treatment
Right to Treatment in the Least Restrictive
   Environment
Right to Refuse Treatment
Right to Aftercare
Client Status and Specific Legal Issues
Voluntary Admissions

Emergency Admissions
Involuntary Admissions
Legal Issues and Special Client Populations
Forensic Clients
   Competency to Stand Trial
   Pleas of Insanity or Mental Illness
Minors
ETHICAL ISSUES IN PSYCHIATRIC–MENTAL HEALTH NURSING CARE
Bioethical Principles in Psychiatric Nursing Practice
Autonomy
Beneficence and Paternalism
Veracity and Fidelity
Justice
Nursing Ethics in Community Mental Health
Boundaries in Ethical Nursing Care

KEY TOPICS

Legal Issues: Nurse practice acts; malpractice and obtaining legal counsel

Basic Rights of Clients Receiving Psychiatric Nursing Care: Informed consent and confidentiality

Evolving Legal Rights: Legal rights to treatment, treatment in the least restrictive environment, refuse treatment, aftercare

Client Status and Specific Legal Issues: Voluntary, emergency, and involuntary admissions

Legal Issues and Special Client Populations: Forensic clients and minors

Ethical Issues in Psychiatric Mental Health Nursing Care

Bioethical Principles: Autonomy; beneficence and paternalism; veracity and fidelity; justice

Nursing Ethics in Community Mental Health

Boundaries in Ethical Nursing Care

■ Exercises

MATCHING

Match the term in Part A with the statement that applies to the term in Part B.

PART A

a. Standards of nursing practice

b. Substituted consent

c. Malpractice

d. Forensic psychiatry

e. Outcome of the Tarasoff v. Board of Regents of Univ. California in 1974

f. Determining factors for the "adequacy of treatment"

g. Respondeat superior

h. Ethics

i. Informed consent

j. Battery

PART B

1. _____ Includes activities such as evaluating competency and mental condition at the time of an alleged crime

2. _____ Written documents that outline minimum expectations for safe nursing care

3. _____ The recipient of health care gives this to treating providers before performing a treatment or procedure.

4. _____ Therapists have a duty to protect a person who is threatened by a client.

5. _____ One example of this is the Health Care Proxy.

6. _____ A tort action that a consumer plaintiff brings against a professional

7. _____ Clients must be treated in a humane environment by qualified staff and with individualized treatment plans.

8. _____ "The acts of employees are attributable to the employer, whom the court will also find responsible for damages to injured third parties."

9. _____ Principles that serve as codes of conduct about right and wrong behaviors

10. _____ Touching another person without his or her consent

SHORT ANSWER

1. Discuss what "the right to least restrictive treatment" means, and explain its importance in psychiatric–mental health nursing.

2. Why was the ruling in the case of "Tarasoff v. Board of Regents of Univ. California in 1974" so important to psychiatry?

3. Think about reasons why it might be difficult to determine an individual's competency to stand trial for murder, and discuss at least two.

CORRECT THE FALSE STATEMENTS

In the statements on the chart, highlight the incorrect portions and restate them in the blank column.

False Statement	Correction
Standards of nursing practice are written documents that explain how and why nurses should deliver excellent, client-centered care.	
The reasonable person test, as applied to the nurse defendant, is a description of the minimum, most reasonable nursing interventions that are required to keep the client safe.	
The application of restraints and the use of seclusion are considered high-risk treatment modalities because they frequently cause psychological trauma, including post-traumatic stress syndrome.	
Paternalism is the same as beneficence, except that the professional defines specific activities and relationships in which the client may engage.	

CRITICAL THINKING AND SELF-EVALUATION EXERCISES

1. Think about a local or national incident when a person has been killed and in which the mental health of the perpetrator has been a consideration.

   a. What are the ethical issues that were operating?

   b. What is your perspective on the perpetrator's guilt or innocence?

   c. How should society deal with perpetrators who are mentally ill?

2. What is your opinion of "assisted suicide"? Under what conditions do you feel it is appropriate, if any? What if the individual who is asking for assistance is mentally ill? Does this change your perceptions?

■ NCLEX-Style Exam Questions

1. Which of the following is the most important reason for psychiatric nurses to understand law, legislation, and legal processes that relate to professional nursing practice?

   a. Because only by lobbying can psychiatric nurses have an impact on the delivery of services on a national level

   b. Because these activities are included in our Code of Ethics

   c. Because doing so gives the nurse the ability to provide quality care that will safeguard the rights and safety of clients

   d. Because doing so gives the nurse guidelines by which to use seclusion and restraint appropriately, when needed

2. Advanced nurse practitioners have:

   a. doctoral degrees.

   b. prescriptive authority in 48 states and get third-party reimbursement in many states.

   c. better financial outcomes than do generalist nurses.

   d. prescriptive authority in 11 states, and are lobbying strongly to win additional states and third-party reimbursement.

3. For a plaintiff to receive monetary damages by suing a professional nurse for malpractice,

he/she must prove all except which of the following elements of nursing negligence?

   a. The nurse professional had a duty of due care toward the plaintiff.

   b. The nurse's performance fell below the standard of care.

   c. The act in which the nurse engaged resulted in physical injury to the client.

   d. The plaintiff consumer must prove his/her injuries.

4. In which of the cases below could the legal theory of "respondeat superior" NOT apply?

   a. If the nurse had contact with and hurt a client in her own home

   b. If the nurse made a medication error that resulted in the client's death

   c. If the nurse slapped a client while running an inpatient group

   d. If the nurse accidentally tripped, fell on an elderly client, and broke the client's hip

5. Which of the following rights could the psychiatric client lose when admitted to a locked, inpatient psychiatric treatment facility?

   a. Right to schedule his or her own time

   b. Right to communicate with an attorney

   c. Right to send and receive mail without censorship

   d. Right to safety from harm

6. A client is admitted for electroconvulsive therapy (ECT). She signed a consent form for this treatment; however, after treatment, she loses her memory. She sues the hospital and staff, stating that the consent form she signed did not include:

   a. risks of treatment.

   b. side effects of treatment.

   c. the way the treatment would be administered.

   d. the prognosis if the treatment or procedure was given.

7. Client charts are legal documents that can be used in court; therefore, all nursing notes and progress records should above all:

   a. provide interpretive, subjective statements by the RN about the client's behavior.

b. include difficulties expressed between professional members of the health care team that may have affected the client's progress.

c. reflect the meaning that the client's behavior had for other clients on the unit.

d. reflect descriptive, nonjudgmental, and objective statements.

8. Dr. Smith, a psychotherapist, hears her client state, "I have had it with this marriage. I'm telling you, and not that I ever would do it, but I feel like hiring a hit man to kill the woman!" Dr. Smith:

a. must warn the client's wife, based on the Tarasoff rule.

b. may be anxious, but since the client did not say he would kill his wife, must hold the client's statements in confidence.

c. is bound to hold all psychotherapeutic content under strict confidence.

d. must keep this confidential, because the client made a disclaimer that he would never do it.

9. Joe, age 70, lives on the street and has become psychotic. On admission to the emergency department, would Joe be admitted even though he has no means to pay his bill?

a. Yes, because it is the ethical responsibility of all health care providers to treat an ill individual.

b. No, because if he has no insurance, the hospital cannot absorb his costs.

c. Yes, because the hospital is bound by law to treat him.

d. No, because his family is in the area, and even though they will not become involved, they are the primary responsible persons.

10. Which of the following is not a client factor in assessment of competency to stand trial?

a. The ability to assist the attorney with defense

b. The ability to understand the nature of the charges filed

c. The ability to relate the sequences of events that led up to the alleged crime

d. The ability to understand courtroom procedures

Working With Individuals

Chapter 8 discusses interventions with the individual client. The client in individual therapy often will work with a team consisting of nurses, a social worker, a psychologist, adjunctive therapists, and a psychiatrist. Psychotherapy is the treatment of mental and emotional disorders using the psychoeducational methods of support, suggestion, persuasion, re-education, reassurance, and insight to alter maladaptive patterns of coping and to encourage personality growth. There are many different types of individual psychotherapy. Cognitive therapy, behavioral therapy, cognitive-behavioral therapy, REBT, choice therapy, and solution-focused therapy are some of the most common types. In addition to listening and observing nonjudgmentally to understand the client's life experience, therapeutic nursing interventions in individual psychiatric nursing care at the basic level include health promotion and health maintenance, intake screening and evaluation, case management, provision of a therapeutic environment (milieu), tracking clients and assisting them with self-care activities, administering and monitoring psychobiological treatment regimens, health teaching, counseling and crisis intervention, psychiatric rehabilitation, community-based care, outreach activities, and advocacy.

LEARNING OBJECTIVES

After completing the exercises in this workbook, and studying the corresponding chapter in the textbook, the student will be able to:

- Define psychotherapy.

- Discuss the collaborative goals of individual therapy.

- Describe various methods or techniques of psychotherapy.

- Compare and contrast the roles of the basic and advanced nurse in individual psychiatric care.

- Discuss therapeutic interventions in nursing.

KEY TERMS

Cognitions: Beliefs and thoughts that color a person's construction of his or her world.

Countertransference: The way that a therapist responds to a client because of feelings the client triggers from the past; a nontherapeutic event that can be resolved with consultation, supervision, or both.

Free association: A technique in which a client says the first thing that comes to his or her mind, without restrictions, in response to something the therapist says.

Negative reinforcement: Removal of an aversive stimulus that results in an increase in behavior or response.

Positive reinforcement: The addition of something that increases the probability of a behavior or response.

Punishment: Presentation of a negative or aversive stimulus or event that results in a decrease in a response or behavior.

Reinforcer: A stimulus that strengthens a new response (behavior) by its repeated association with that response.

Schema or core beliefs: An accumulation of the person's learning and experience within the family, religion, ethnicity, gender, regional subgroups, and broader society.

Structural and functional analysis: An assessment of the functional relationships between various purported motivational variables and the rate of occurrence of certain behaviors.

Transference: The unconscious reenactment of relationship patterns and feelings from the client's past, in which there is distortion of the therapist's behaviors and then an unconscious placing of positive or negative feelings about the situation or person on the therapist.

Chapter Outline

TYPES OF INDIVIDUAL PSYCHOTHERAPY
Classic Psychoanalysis
Cognitive Therapy
Issues Identified by Cognitive Therapy
  Cognitive Triad
  Cognitive Distortion
  Schema or Core Beliefs (Basic Rules of Life)
Cognitive Therapy Treatment Approach
Behavioral Therapy
Behavioral Theory
The Process of Behavioral Therapy
Cognitive-Behavioral Therapy
Rational Emotive Behavior Therapy
Choice Therapy
Brief, Solution-Focused Therapy
THE NURSE'S ROLE
Levels of Clinical Nursing Practice
Therapeutic Interventions in Nursing
Health Promotion and Health Maintenance
Intake Screening and Evaluation
Case Management
Assisting with Self-Care Activities
Implementing Psychobiological Interventions
Health Teaching
Counseling and Crisis Intervention
Psychiatric Rehabilitation

KEY TOPICS

Individual psychotherapy: Many types; several are appropriate for nurses at the basic and advanced levels

Nursing role in individual psychotherapy: Basic and advanced levels of practice merit different nursing roles; therapeutic interventions for the basic-level psychiatric–mental health nurse include, for example, health teaching, case management, intake screening, and health promotion activities.

■ Exercises

MATCHING

Match the term in Part A with the statement that best applies to the term in Part B.

PART A

a. classic psychoanalysis

b. advanced practice psychiatric nurse

c. psychobiological interventions

d. countertransference

e. psychiatric rehabilitation

f. generalist psychiatric nurse

g. cognitive triad

h. behavioral theory

i. cognitive therapy

j. choice therapy

PART B

1. _____ Often consults with psychiatrist on which medications to prescribe for the client

2. _____ Relaxation techniques, nutrition and diet management, exercise and rest schedules

3. _____ Involves exploring the client's conscious and unconscious conflicts and coping behaviors

4. _____ Focuses on the here and now, with the present as the only reality to consider

5. _____ Based on the early stimulus/response research of Pavlov

6. _____ The client's negative view of self, the world, and the future

7. _____ May incorporate principles from different psychotherapeutic techniques into their general interactions with clients, but they will not function as individual therapists

8. _____ Focus is strengthening self-care and promoting and improving the quality of an individual's life through relapse prevention.

9. _____ The client reminds his therapist of her father, who was very abusive.

10. _____ Is based on the premise that the way a person perceives an event, rather than the event itself, determines its relevance

CASE STUDY

John R. was admitted to your psychiatric inpatient unit with the diagnosis of major depressive disorder. He had moved in with his older brother, who had sexually abused John when he was 15 years old. His brother reports that John had begun to stay up all night and sleep all day. He had recently placed a sign on his door saying, "No one need enter...there is no life here." His brother became concerned and brought him into the psychiatric emergency department. The ER assessment includes the following: weight loss of 20 lb in the past month, frequent crying, sleep cycle disturbance, suicidal ideations, and withdrawal from all contact.

When you see John, he is sitting with his head down and does not make eye contact with you. At one point, John states that he is a "horrible husband" and that "It seems that nothing ever goes my way." During your assessment interview, John perks up slightly and is able to look at you occasionally. He cries frequently, stating, "My life is a mess, and my entire world is upside down! I really can't see a future for myself."

1. John evidences components of the "cognitive triad" identified by Beck. List the three components of this triad, and add specific data that would support your assessment.

2. Using what you have learned in Chapter 8, complete the table by (a) naming two theories (with theorist) of individual psychotherapy that may be useful with John; (b) describing how each of these theorists might explain John's symptoms; and (c) designing at least two nursing interventions using this theoretical approach. You may add data that will support your ideas (eg, that John is gay). An example is provided in the first row.

CRITICAL THINKING AND SELF-EVALUATION EXERCISES

Think about your own philosophy of nursing. Which of the theories that were presented in this chapter best matches your own philosophy? List some nursing interventions that you would be more likely to be comfortable with and some that you would be less comfortable with, given your philosophy and its relationship to a given theory.

Theory/Theorist	How Theorist Might Explain John's Symptoms	Nursing Interventions Based On Theoretical Base
Classic Psychoanalysis (Freud)	John is suffering from a breakdown in his defense mechanisms. This may be caused by the fact that he is living with his brother. The intimacy of living with the perpetrator of his abuse serves to crumble his normal defenses, such as intellectualization, rationalization, and repression.	During the first 2 days of care, the RN will: 1. Establish trust with John 2. Identify, with John, defense mechanisms that have eroded 3. Work with John to understand the connection between his current hospitalization and moving in with his brother

NCLEX-Style Exam Questions

1. Of the following, which treatment modalities have the greatest empirical support?
   a. Classic psychoanalysis and behavioral therapy
   b. Behavioral therapy and choice therapy
   c. Cognitive therapy and behavioral therapy
   d. Motivational therapy and classic psychoanalysis

2. One of the biggest differences between psychiatric nursing and medical–surgical nursing is that:
   a. psychiatric nurses focus only on the psychological aspects, whereas medical–surgical nurses focus on the physiological.
   b. psychiatric nurses facilitate clients' identification of resources and use of personal resources to get what they need, and medical–surgical nurses do many more things for clients.
   c. generalist-level medical–surgical nurses are educated in the biological aspects of body functioning, whereas generalists in psychiatric–mental health nursing are educated more in the psychological aspects.
   d. medical–surgical nurses often avoid dealing with the client's emotional difficulties, focusing rather on the task at hand, whereas psychiatric nurses rarely focus on tasks.

3. Of the following, which is *not* a type of individual therapy?
   a. Psychoanalysis
   b. Behavioral
   c. Cognitive
   d. Deconstructional

4. Jodie is an RN whose client reminds her of her sister, with whom she has a close and positive relationship. This phenomenon is best characterized by which term?
   a. Transference
   b. Free association
   c. Countertransference
   d. Reaction formation

5. A cognitive therapist would say that there are three issues that result in the formation and maintenance of common psychological disorders. All but which of the following are in that list?
   a. Cognitive triad
   b. Cognitive denial
   c. Cognitive distortion
   d. Schema or core beliefs

6. All except which of the following are cognitive therapy techniques?
   a. Reviewing homework assignments
   b. Listing an agenda for each session
   c. Listing primary defenses used in life
   d. Reviewing the session prior to ending

7. Some behavioral therapists believe that seclusion and restraint are forms of punishment. You may assume that these therapists view seclusion and restraint as:
   a. a treatment administered only when all others have failed.
   b. an unpleasant stimulus that happens after a certain unwanted behavior.
   c. continuous negative reinforcement for a response.
   d. an unavoidable consequence of aberrant behaviors.

8. How would Ellis describe a rational belief?
   a. An evaluative cognition that is expressed as a wish, like, and dislike that may or may not be attained
   b. The belief that humans can change their thinking no matter what the circumstances
   c. A belief that is grounded in the individual's past experience with the family of origin
   d. A belief that makes sense to most of the normal population

9. A generalist psychiatric nurse works with his client to uncover a past abuse that the nurse learned about from the client's mother (not the client). Which of the following best describes this nurse's intervention?
   a. The generalist is working outside his scope of practice and should not be doing this intervention.

b. The generalist is concerned about the client and is implementing a treatment of choice in this situation.

c. The generalist should have ignored the data he received from this client's mother, because it has no relation to the current hospitalization.

d. The generalist is operating under the concept of beneficence.

10. All but which of the following are areas of focus within psychiatric rehabilitation?

a. Consumer empowerment

b. Emphasis on recovery of hope and of function

c. Stronger collaborative relationships with treatment services

d. Reduction in acute symptoms of psychosis

Working With Groups

Chapter 9 will identify and discuss concepts related to the treatment of clients in groups. A group is three or more people with related goals; groups vary according to their size, homogeneity of membership, climate, norms, and goal directedness. Styles of group leadership, important concepts of group communication, and stages of group development will be discussed. The advantages of group therapy include its effectiveness and efficiency in time and cost. Therapeutic factors are elements observed in group therapy that are the basis for client change and growth in groups. Most therapeutic group experiences can be categorized as psychotherapy or growth groups. Nurses participate as leaders and co-leaders in multiple formal and informal groups; contemporary nursing groups are influenced by social and societal needs. Examples include intergenerational groups, medication noncompliance groups, and coping skills groups.

LEARNING OBJECTIVES

After completing the exercises in this workbook, and studying the corresponding chapter in the textbook, the student will be able to:

- Identify the characteristics of a group.

- Explain group norms.

- Compare styles of group leadership.

- Define three major categories of group roles.

- Identify communication processes within groups.

- Describe the stages of group development.

- Discuss the advantages of group therapy.

- Discuss the therapeutic factors of group therapy.

- Compare the various types of group therapy.

- Discuss the nurse's role in working with groups.

KEY TERMS

Autocratic leader: A leader who exercises significant authority and control over group members, rarely if ever seeks or uses input from the group, and does not encourage participation or interaction from the group.

Democratic leader: A leader who encourages group interaction and participation in group problem-solving and decision-making, values the input and feedback of each group member, seeks spontaneous and honest interaction among group members, creates an atmosphere that rewards members for their contributions, solicits the group's opinions, and tailors the group's work to their common goals.

Formal group: A group with structure and authority, which usually emanates from above; interaction in the group is usually limited.

Group: Three or more people with related goals.

Group norm: The development, over time, of a pattern of interaction within a group to which certain behavioral expectations are attached.

Informal group: A group that provides much of a person's education and contributes greatly to his or her cultural values; members do not depend on one another.

Laissez-faire leader: A leader who allows group members to operate as they choose.

Power: The perceived ability to control appropriate reward, therefore lending influence.

Primary group: A group that has face-to-face contact, boundaries, norms, and explicit and implicit interdependent roles.

Secondary group: A group that usually is larger and more impersonal than a primary group; members do not have the relationship bonds or emotional ties of members of a primary group.

Chapter Outline

KEY TOPICS

Groups as a modality for therapeutic treatment: Leadership styles, group communication, stages of group development, advantages of group therapy, and therapeutic factors

Psychiatric nursing role in groups: Group process and therapy in nursing education and practice

■ Exercises

MATCHING

Match the term in Part A with the statement that applies to the term in Part B.

PART A

a. autocratic leadership

b. group norm

c. group roles

d. group

e. content and process

f. formal group

g. transference

h. characteristics of groups

i. working stage of group

j. laissez-faire leaders

PART B

1. _____ Three or more people with related goals

2. _____ What is being said and how the group handles communication

3. _____ When a client attributes characteristics of a family member/significant other to the therapist

4. _____ The real work of the group is accomplished; conflict and cooperation surface

5. _____ Style that imposes authority and control over group members

6. _____ Size, homogeneity, stability, cohesiveness, climate, conformity to norms

7. _____ An interactional pattern that has certain behaviors that are expected; develops over time

8. _____ Chiefs of Staff for the President; a group with structure and authority

9. _____ Group task, group building, group maintenance

10. _____ Usually allow group members to do what they choose in the group

GROUP COMMUNICATION TECHNIQUE EXERCISE

Fill in the accompanying technique chart, using new examples from your own ideas.
Avoid using examples from the textbook.

Technique	Define/Describe	Give An Example
SILENCE		
INTERVENTION		
REASSURANCE		
APPROVAL		
ACCEPTANCE		
CLARIFICATION		
IDENTIFICATION		
INTERPRETATION		

SHORT ANSWER

You are leading a health education group for clients in an acute psychiatric hospital. For each of the following group stages in the chart provided, fill in the goal of the stage, and then give examples of how you, as the group leader, would facilitate work during this phase of group development.

Stage	Goal	Leadership Interventions You Would Use
INITIAL		
WORKING		
MATURE		
TERMINATION		

CRITICAL THINKING AND SELF-EVALUATION EXERCISES

Think about a group you have been in recently, and answer the following questions:

1. Was this an informal or formal group?

2. What was the style of leadership in this group?

3. How did you feel about being in this group? Why?

4. Did the group accomplish its goals? Why or why not?

5. Do you enjoy being in groups, or would you rather do things alone? Why?

■ NCLEX-Style Exam Questions

1. Which of the following statements would indicate that the group is in the working phase of development?

   a. "Let's go around the circle and tell one thing that you enjoy doing."

   b. "What have you learned, and how will you take this out into your life?"

   c. "I don't understand why Mary doesn't see my point of view, and frankly it really irritates me when she does that!"

   d. "I'm not sure what we are supposed to be talking about."

2. Which of the following group characteristics is reflective of the statement: "Our group never talks about really emotional issues . . . I mean, no one ever cries."
   a. Group homogeneity
   b. Group stability
   c. Conformity to group norms
   d. Group climate

3. When the group is attempting to determine a time and place for meetings, Shaundra, the leader, states, "We can discuss when it is best for most members, and then find a place that you would be comfortable with." This demonstrates which of the leadership styles below?
   a. Laissez-faire
   b. Autocratic
   c. Naturalistic
   d. Democratic

4. Which of the group roles listed below is best reflected by the client who consistently validates members' contributions, tries to be the "mediator" between members, and interprets the group's procedures?
   a. Group building and maintenance role
   b. Individual role
   c. Task role
   d. Group cohesion role

5. The initiator-contributor, information seeker, information giver, and coordinator are examples of which of the following?
   a. Group building roles
   b. Individual roles
   c. Task roles
   d. Group cohesion roles

6. A client, John, has been talking to another client, Marcy, about her frequent denial in group for 2 weeks. On the third week, Marcy comes late to group. When they begin to discuss her lateness, Marcy gets up and leaves. The content of this exchange is the discussion. The process that is occurring may be:

   a. Marcy is angry with John for his confrontation.
   b. John is taking out his frustrations on himself.
   c. other group members are not very strong.
   d. the group leader is not meeting John's dependency needs.

7. The following statements are heard in a group: "You can't say that because you don't really know me." "I wonder if the therapist is going to leave?" and "I'm not sure whether or not I can really talk freely." These best reflect which of the following group themes?
   a. Guilt and punishment
   b. Fear for safety
   c. Trust and belonging
   d. Loss and abandonment

8. The working stage of group therapy is marked by:
   a. members' propensity to leave the group.
   b. conflict and cooperation among group members.
   c. therapists' tendency to "back off" to allow the group to work.
   d. group members' concern about confidentiality issues.

9. All except which of the following are therapeutic factors identified by Yalom?
   a. universality
   b. regulation
   c. altruism
   d. existentialism

10. The oldest and best-known therapeutic method that came out of the sensitivity training group movement was the:
    a. encounter group.
    b. T group.
    c. growth group.
    d. psychotherapy group.

CHAPTER 10

Working With Families

In the past 150 years, Americans with mental illness have been "to the asylum and back." The result is that their families are again their primary caregivers. Nurses work with the families of those with psychiatric disorders for two purposes: to help them cope with the traumatic effects of mental illness and caregiving and to involve them as allies in their ill relatives' treatments.

Stigma and discrimination (in housing, employment, and insurance coverage) as well as confidentiality laws and involuntary commitment laws are sources of individual and family burden. The family members of persons with a serious mental illness are a population at risk for genetically linked mental illnesses, stress-related medical disorders and social problems, or both.

Family consultation designed to reduce family burden is a prime example of a needed secondary prevention strategy. Nurses functioning as family consultants mentor families, meaning they provide information, advice, and support about mental illness and caregiving. Effective communication with families is clear and respectful and based on the assumption (unless proven otherwise) that families are doing their best and have the client's best interests at heart. Although most family members' needs are met by nonclinical services (support and education), a minority (including caregivers who are also clients) need clinical services (psychotherapy, marriage counseling, and medication). Family advocacy organizations such as NAMI and DMDA are excellent resources for family and professional caregivers.

LEARNING OBJECTIVES

After completing the exercises in this workbook, and studying the corresponding chapter in the textbook, the student will be able to:

- Trace the history of family caregiving in the United States from 1850 to 2000.

- Explain the rationale for involving families in clients' treatment.

- Define family burden.

- Differentiate among objective, subjective, and iatrogenic burden.

- Define *family resilience*.

- Describe a resilient family.

- Explain secondary prevention and its relevance to working with families who have a relative with a serious mental illness.

- Explain *family consultation* and how it differs from family therapy.

- Provide examples of how nurses can function as family consultants.

- Differentiate between family psychoeducation and family education.

- Refer families to local support, educational, and advocacy services available from NAMI and DMDA.

KEY TERMS

Deinstitutionalization: The massive discharge of clients from state hospitals that began in the 1950s, accelerated in the 1960s and 1970s, and continues today as psychiatric treatment continues to move from inpatient to outpatient settings.

Depressive/Manic Depressive Association (DMDA): A national support and advocacy association with regional chapters for people with depressive and bipolar disorders and their families.

Families: In this chapter, used to mean families with a relative who has a serious mental illness.

Family burden: The effects of serious mental illness on the family (see iatrogenic burden, objective burden, and subjective burden).

Family consultation: A professional service offered to families to reduce family burden; a type of secondary prevention, originally called supportive counseling.

Family education: Educational programs of varying duration to increase family members' knowledge about mental illness, caregiving, and self-care, with the objective of improving the entire family's quality of life.

Family member: In this chapter, used to mean the parent, sibling, offspring, or spouse of a person with a serious mental illness.

Family psychoeducation: A lengthy educational program for families (including the client) that is team-taught by professionals and includes, in addition to didactic content about mental illness, extensive training in behavioral skills intended to create a home environment conducive to reducing relapse and recidivism.

Family resilience: The family's capacity to rebound from the effects of mental illness.

Family support services: Opportunities for mutual support available without cost to families through groups organized by family organizations (e.g., NAMI, DMDA).

Iatrogenic burden: From the Greek *iatros* (physician) and *iasthai* (to heal). Used here to mean family burden exacerbated by the mental health system or mental health professionals.

NAMI, The Nation's Voice on Mental Illness: Formerly known as the National Alliance for the Mentally Ill, a national advocacy organization with state and local affiliates dedicated to improving the lives of persons with serious mental illness and their families.

Objective burden: The practical problems associated with caregiving (e.g., employment issues, financial drain).

Secondary prevention: An intervention to prevent further damage after a traumatic event; in this context, interventions to prevent families subjected to the trauma of mental illness from experiencing further adverse consequences (e.g., caregiver burnout, disrupted interpersonal relationships, psychiatric and medical health problems).

Serious mental illness: A term given to a psychiatric disorder that meets the criteria for duration (at least 1 year), disability (relatively severe functional impairment), and diagnosis (including schizophrenia, bipolar disorder, and major depression) (National Advisory Mental Health Council, 1993).

Subjective burden: The emotional response the client and family have to mental illness and caregiving (e.g., grief, fear, guilt, anger). (Some researchers define subjective burden differently, as *perceived* objective burden.)

Chapter Outline

FAMILY CAREGIVING 1850 TO 2000
FAMILY BURDEN
Objective Burden
Subjective Burden

Iatrogenic Burden
Confidentiality Issues
Involuntary Treatment Statutes
Discrimination
Burden Attributable to Professionals
FAMILY RESILIENCE
NEEDS OF FAMILIES FOR SECONDARY PREVENTION
Families as a Population at Risk
Family Consultation
Family Consultation Versus Family Therapy
Components of Family Consultation
The Nurse as Family Consultant
Family Empowerment
Family Education
Family Education Versus Family Psychoeducation
Components of Family Education
The Nurse as Family Educator
Peer-Taught Family Education
Psychotherapy and Medication

KEY TOPICS

Family caregiving: Family burden, family resilience

Family needs for secondary prevention: Families as populations at risk; family consultation, empowerment, and education; psychotherapy and medication

■ Exercises

MATCHING

Match the term in Part A with the statement that applies to the term in Part B.

PART A

a. objective family burden

b. family empowerment

c. family resiliency

d. family education

e. NAMI

f. family consultation

g. family psychoeducation

h. subjective family burden

i. family therapy

j. iatrogenic burden

PART B

1. _____ The act of supporting family members' sense of self-worth and sense of control

2. _____ Practical problems family members face while caring for ill relatives

3. _____ The mentorship and support of families to expand their knowledge and help them to access support organizations

4. _____ The characteristic that families have wherein the mental illness in a member acts as a catalyst for positive change

5. _____ Designed to advocate nationally for needs of the mentally ill and their families

6. _____ Negative emotions that family members experience in response to a loved one's mental illness

7. _____ An intervention in which the mentally ill family member has historically been viewed as the "symptom bearer" for a disturbed family system, and signals pain for the whole family

8. _____ Provision of materials and information about mental illness to family members

9. _____ Experiences of family members of attitudes and behaviors of some mental health professionals who cling to outmoded theories about families

10. _____ Providing the family with extensive training in communication and behavioral skills

TIME LINE EXERCISE

Label eight large index cards or sheets of heavy paper with the following dates: 1848, 1850s, 1950s, 1955, 1963, 1979, 1999, Present. On each card, indicate the prevailing philosophies about family involvement in treatment of the mentally ill, any individuals who made a difference in influencing social change in this area, treatment environments of the mentally ill individual, and the family's level of participation in care. Bring the cards to class, and post them on the board in a timeline. Synthesize information obtained into one comprehensive time-line that will illustrate the progression of the inclusion of families in mental health care.

CASE STUDY

John has had schizophrenia for 2 years. He is living with his parents, Susan and Lloyd Weid, because they recently found him walking in the street in their small town, disheveled and penniless. The family is a lower-middle-class family, and they have two other teenagers at home. Taking John in has caused turmoil in the family. They have been faced with transporting John to his psychiatric appointments, getting his medications, taking care of his food and laundry, and trying to include him in family activities. John's parents have struggled recently with feelings of anger that John is causing such a disruption in their family life. They also fear that he will not be able to be on his own, and they grieve over the loss of the "healthy" child that they raised. They have guilt that they even have these feelings, as well as guilt because of how John is also disrupting the lives of his younger siblings, who often complain bitterly to the couple. Susan, John's mother, has begun staying up late at night ruminating about the situation, crying frequently, and is losing weight. Lloyd tries to be the "strong" one and is supportive of Susan; however, his work at a local furniture company frequently takes him out of the house during the evenings, as he works the night shift. This leaves Susan with the task of managing John and her other two teens in the evenings, which is a very difficult time for her. After a month of managing John on their own, the Weids went with John to his therapist, asking for help. The therapist stated that there were no supportive services in their small midwestern town, but that she would refer the couple to the closest case management service she knew of, in a large city approximately 200 miles from their home. She also stated that since John had developed his problems within the home setting, it might be best for him to try and resolve them in the same place. The couple left feeling disheartened, unsupported, and hopeless.

1. Describe the types of family burden being experienced by the Weid family.

2. Define "population at risk" and explain how this family might be viewed as being "at risk." Include potential health, psychological, and social risks.

3. If the Weids had been referred to you for a family consultation, define how you could intervene, using the "Three F" approach.

4. What might you do to help empower this family?

5. What are the Weids' needs in regard to family education, and how would you help them get these needs met?

5. Which of the family members appears to be more at risk and would benefit from a full assessment of symptoms?

CRITICAL THINKING AND SELF-EVALUATION EXERCISES

1. Have you ever had the experience of a family member being seriously ill, with any type of illness (medical or psychiatric)? If so, describe your feelings about this at that time.

2. What feelings did you experience when you heard that your loved one was ill?

3. List some ideas about what you would have liked to receive in terms of support from health care providers.

■ NCLEX-Style Exam Questions

1. The goal of the deinstitutionalization movement was to:
   a. move psychiatric clients out of the hospitals and into the community in an effort to provide a better quality of life for them.
   b. move psychiatric clients out of the hospitals and into their families of origin, because of the belief that families were the responsible parties.
   c. move chronic, older psychiatric clients out of hospitals in order to make room for younger clients who had better prognoses and were amenable to long-term treatment.
   d. empty out large psychiatric hospitals so they could be converted for military use.

2. Many families take years to understand that a member is mentally ill and to identify the warning signs of relapse. During this period, they try to normalize puzzling behaviors. This is called:
   a. avoidance.
   b. ignorance.
   c. reaction formation.
   d. denial.

3. The Taylor family is struggling to make ends meet since their 28-year-old daughter, Joanie, came to live with them. Joanie has bipolar disorder and requires frequent supervision and assistance with her ADLs, money management, and transportation. The Taylors are experiencing:
   a. subjective family burden.
   b. objective family burden.
   c. iatrogenic family burden.
   d. general family burden.

4. Today, which of the following health care providers are specially trained to take the responsibility of helping clients with multiple services, such as money management, transportation, ADL assistance, and crisis intervention?
   a. The generalist psychiatric nurse
   b. The advanced-level psychiatric nurse
   c. The case manager
   d. The social worker

5. The Lawson family has been caring for Randy, their 35-year-old son with schizophrenia, for about 15 years. They report that they often are fearful that Randy will become psychotic and hurt someone in public. They are sad because they remember that when Randy was in high school, he was a star student and athlete, and they enjoyed watching him play football. These feelings of the family can best be described as:
   a. inability to cope with the difficult work of caring for Randy.
   b. exaggerated response to a normal, manageable situation.
   c. subjective family burden that occurs in many families who have a mentally ill loved one.
   d. objective family burden that includes many thoughts and feelings about caring for a loved one who is psychotic.

6. Why have NAMI family member professionals been advocating for change in the preservice training programs of nursing and other professions since 1980?
   a. Treatments that were taught in these programs changed drastically each year.
   b. The content that was taught about the etiology of mental illnesses often revolved around the family's role in illness onset.
   c. The content included biological approaches to the etiology of mental illness, which we know are not founded in research.

d. NAMI was concerned about the notion that educators had not had any formal experiences or training in psychiatry.

7. When the Sorenson family realized that their daughter, Emily, was severely depressed, they accompanied her to the therapist. There, they learned about major depression, the medications that are used, and symptom management. Emily's depression resulted in the family's rallying around her and created a climate in the family of support and strength. This phenomenon is best described as:

a. iatrogenic coping.

b. subjective burden relief.

c. family cross-relief.

d. resiliency.

8. Working with families who have a mentally ill loved one falls into which category?

a. Primary prevention

b. Secondary prevention

c. Tertiary prevention

d. Quaternary prevention

9. Why are families with a mentally ill member considered to be an "at-risk population"?

a. A younger sibling often mimics the behavior of the mentally ill older sibling, which can be dangerous.

b. The mentally ill member can be dangerous at times, often risking loss of property and home.

c. They often experience caregiver burnout, stress-related health problems, depression, and anxiety, which call for family intervention.

d. Family members often become angry and are at risk for harming others either physically or psychologically.

10. Which of the following is *not* included in the "Three F" approach to family consultation?

a. Feeling

b. Forgiving

c. Focus

d. Finding

Working With Special Environments: Forensic Clients, Crisis Intervention, and the Homeless

Chapter 11 explores the role of the psychiatric nurse in special environments, including forensics, crisis intervention, and homelessness. Forensic psychiatric nursing helps to bridge the gap between the criminal justice system and the mental health care system. Forensic settings include forensic psychiatric facilities, locked units of general hospitals, and state hospitals.

Crisis intervention differs from traditional psychotherapy primarily because it focuses on the here-and-now and immediate problem-solving. Nurses are often the first health care professionals in contact with the client in crisis; therefore, they are uniquely positioned to intervene in crisis.

The homeless population is heterogeneous and encompasses the young, older adults, families with children, victims of domestic violence, street youth, veterans, those released from jails, immigrants, and the mentally ill. Shelters and programs for the homeless are crucial, but they do not offer the solution to the deeper structural problems of poverty, inadequate housing, and prejudice toward the mentally ill.

The role of the nurse is crucial in identifying and removing barriers to care, providing fair and thorough assessments, and providing quality care to those who are so alienated on the margins of society that they are incapable of using the traditional mental health system.

LEARNING OBJECTIVES

After completing the exercises in this workbook, and studying the corresponding chapter in the textbook, the student will be able to:

- Describe the nurse's role in the forensic milieu.

- Describe characteristics of and health concerns specific to the forensic population, addressing implications for nursing care.

- Apply the nursing process to care of clients in forensic settings.

- Discuss the development phases of crisis theory.

- Differentiate maturational, situational, and adventitious crises.

- Discuss the goals and methods of crisis intervention.

- Apply the nursing process to a client or family in crisis.

- Discuss crisis intervention as a component of case management, psychosocial rehabilitation, and managed care.

- Identify current trends in the homeless population.

- Discuss factors that contribute to homelessness in the mentally ill population.

- Discuss barriers that prevent homeless mentally ill persons from receiving care, and measures to promote their access.

- Describe specific health care concerns of homeless mentally ill people.

- Apply the nursing process to the care of homeless mentally ill clients.

KEY TERMS

Adventitious crisis: A crisis precipitated by an unexpected event (e.g., natural disaster, bombing, mass shooting).

Crisis intervention: Methods and techniques used to assist a person in distress to resolve the immediate problem and regain emotional equilibrium.

Expressive violence: Interpersonal violence, usually between people known to one another and of similar age, ethnicity, and cultural background.

Gang violence: Violence associated with group membership and committed for retaliation or revenge (see Chapter 11 text references: Labecki, 1994; Sigler, 1995).

Instrumental violence: Violent acts that are usually premeditated and motive-driven (frequently economic gain), usually involving people unknown to one another.

Maturational or developmental crisis: A crisis precipitated by the normal stress of development.

Situational crisis: A crisis precipitated by a sudden traumatic event (e.g., job loss).

Chapter Outline

FORENSIC NURSING
Forensic Settings
Factors Contributing to Incarceration
Characteristics of the Forensic Population
Mentally Ill Offenders
Violent Offenders
Special Populations
  Juvenile Offenders
  Female Offenders
  Older Adult Offenders
  Minority Offenders
  Offenders with HIV, AIDS, or Hepatitis
Effects of Incarceration on Mental Health
Characteristics of Forensic Psychiatric Nurses
Attitudes
Skills
APPLICATION OF THE NURSING PROCESS TO THE FORENSIC CLIENT
Assessment
Content
Risk of Suicide
Nursing Diagnosis
Planning
Implementation
Promoting Health
Maintaining an Interdisciplinary Approach to Care
Focusing on the Family
Ensuring Continuity of Care
Acting as an Advocate
Evaluation
NURSING CARE FOR THE CLIENT IN CRISIS
Crisis Theory
Phases of a Crisis
Types of Crises
  Maturational Crisis
  Situational Crisis
  Adventitious Crisis
Crisis Prevention
Crisis Intervention and Stabilization
Crisis Intervention Versus Traditional Therapies
Crisis Intervention Across Contexts
Characteristics and Skills of the Crisis Intervener
Crisis Intervention Variations
  Team Approach
  Crisis Groups
  Families in Crisis
  Telephone Counseling

APPLICATION OF THE NURSING PROCESS TO THE CLIENT IN CRISIS
Assessment
Evaluating Feelings
Determining Perception of the Event
Assessing Support Systems
Assessing Coping Skills
Determining Potential for Self-Harm
Nursing Diagnosis
Planning
Implementation
Realizing the Potential for Growth
Learning to Ask for Help
Using Adaptive Coping
Focusing on Problem Resolution
Using Information Technology
Evaluation
NURSING CARE OF HOMELESS CLIENTS
Demographics
Homeless Mentally Ill People
Factors Contributing to Homelessness in the Mentally Ill
  Lack of Prevention
  Functional Abilities and Deficits
  Poverty
  Inadequate Housing
  Substance Abuse
  High Mobility
Critical Issues Affecting the Homeless Mentally Ill
  A Changing Mental Health System
  Barriers to Care
  The Shelter System
  Health Concerns
  The Criminal Justice System

KEY TOPICS

Forensic Nursing: Forensic settings; characteristics of forensic populations and of forensic nurses; factors contributing to incarceration; effects of incarceration on mental health; nursing process in forensic nursing

Crisis Intervention: Phases and theories of crisis intervention; types of crises; prevention; intervention and stabilization; the nursing process in crisis intervention

Homelessness: Demographics; factors contributing to homelessness; the homeless mentally ill and factors affecting this group

■ Exercises

MATCHING

Match the term in Part A with the statement that applies to the term in Part B.

PART A

a. adventitious crisis

b. situational crisis

c. crisis

d. crisis intervention

e. barriers to care

f. maturational crisis

g. expressive violence

h. factors influencing outcomes of crisis

i. gang violence

j. instrumental violence

PART B

1. _____ Interpersonal violence

2. _____ Usually premeditated and motive-driven, involving people who do not know each other

3. _____ Perception of the problem, help or hindrance from significant others, previous problem-solving experience

4. _____ Precipitated by an unexpected event

5. _____ Violence associated with group membership, committed for retaliation or revenge

6. _____ Methods used to help persons in distress to resolve the immediate problem and to regain equilibrium

7. _____ Precipitated by a sudden, traumatic event

8. _____ A turning point in which the person is unsure what to do

9. _____ Precipitated by the normal stress of development

10. _____ Lack of insurance, lack of transportation, fear and concern about scrutiny

CORRECT THE FALSE STATEMENTS

In the sentences below, circle and replace incorrect words with the correct ones.

1. Currently, Poland has the highest incarceration rate in the Western world.

   _____

2. Forensic clients often demonstrate poor judgment, limited but available family support, limited reasoning abilities, and exceptionally high levels of anxiety disorders.

   _____

3. Instrumental violence is associated with group membership and is usually done for revenge or retaliation for a perceived wrong.

   _____

4. Forensic psychiatric nurses are often secure in their roles, and have dual obligations: one of social necessity and social good and one of maintaining safety in the jail facility.

   _____

5. In forensic settings, the incidence of self-violence and suicide is much lower than in the general population because of the extreme, 24-hour monitoring systems in place.

   _____

6. The active crisis state is long-term, usually lasting at least 3 months.

   _____

7. The first phase of a crisis is marked by anxiety caused by the failure of usual coping mechanisms; the second phase includes anxiety in response to a trauma; the third phase involves the inadequacy of the person's inner resources and supports; and the fourth is marked by escalating anxiety.

   _____

8. Melody was in a building when the roof caved in next to her. She becomes depressed and anxious, reflecting the onset of a developmental crisis.

   _____

9. Crisis intervention differs from traditional therapies in that it focuses more on the individual's past experiences and their relationship to current events.

_____

10. Black men are the primary group that can be found in homeless shelters, although white couples are increasingly being found in shelters in large cities.

_____

11. Research has shown that the homeless mentally ill account for 85% of the homeless population, and that over 70% of the total homeless population demonstrate symptoms of anxiety.

_____

12. Common contributing factors to homelessness include lack of mental health care, poor work ethics, anergia, inadequate supportive housing, avolition, and the stigma and discrimination associated with mental illness.

_____

13. Major goals for a homeless mentally ill person include: (a) client will satisfy physical needs and remain safe; (b) client will engage in educational opportunities to establish experience for employment; (c) client will identify and use psychosocial supports; and (d) client will report to therapist every 2 weeks, minimally.

_____

CRITICAL THINKING AND SELF-EVALUATION EXERCISES

1. Imagine yourself being homeless. Given your current situation (location, environment, weather, etc.), describe how you might live.

2. What would your major concerns be as a homeless person?

3. Imagine that you are on the street and are panhandling to get money for food. How would it feel to look up into the eyes of a passerby?

4. Have you ever walked past a homeless person (ie, a "street person" or "bag lady")? What were your initial thoughts, and what did you think about that person?

■ NCLEX-Style Exam Questions

1. All except which of the following are common factors contributing to incarceration?
   a. Increased illegal drug-related activities
   b. Criminalization of the mentally ill
   c. Anticrime legislation
   d. Recession in the economy

2. Forensic clients have complex issues. Which of the following is a factor to consider when working with this population?
   a. Prevalence of mental disorder
   b. Ability to understand the language
   c. Level of education attained
   d. Sexual preference

3. Joe and Mark are two black males, aged 28, who are roommates. They have recently been arguing over a mutual female friend, and one night Mark impulsively shoots Joe with a gun they keep in the kitchen for protection. Which type of violence is being displayed?
   a. Expressive
   b. Instrumental
   c. Gang
   d. Mutual

4. One of the most difficult challenges faced by forensic psychiatric nurses is:
   a. balancing the dual obligations of caring for clients and meeting social expectations.
   b. deciding how and when to leave the field and return to hospital or community-based nursing.
   c. protecting themselves from violence perpetrated by their clients.
   d. maintaining boundaries between themselves and incarcerated clients and their families.

5. In caring for the forensic client, a barrier to the nursing assessment process includes:
   a. physical environment and lack of privacy.
   b. inability to speak with the client directly.
   c. being left alone in a room without adequate supervision for the client.
   d. anxiety of the nurse related to being in a jail facility.

6. Crisis theory holds that an imbalance exists between the client's problem and the immediate resources available to deal with it. Which of the following best describes the active crisis state?

   a. It lasts about 4–6 weeks.

   b. It lasts for 2–3 months if left untreated.

   c. It is a pathological response to a normal problem.

   d. It is often remedied by the appropriate medication.

7. The response to crisis has been analyzed by Hoff, who divided it into four areas. Which of the following is *not* one of Hoff's areas of crisis response?

   a. Feelings

   b. Thoughts and perceptions

   c. Family responses

   d. Biophysical responses

8. In assessing a homeless person, the psychiatric nurse faces many obstacles. When a homeless client asks to meet the nurse in a local coffee shop rather than at the shelter where he lives, what is the best therapeutic response for the nurse?

   a. "Although I see you want to do that, I really think we need to stay in your day-to-day environment."

   b. "No, that's not possible, because it is outside your local area."

   c. "I would feel uncomfortable doing that. Let's stay here."

   d. "It sounds as though meeting in the shelter would be uncomfortable for you. Can you tell me more about your feelings?"

9. Why would the psychiatric nurse need to be cautious about formulating nursing diagnoses quickly for a homeless person?

   a. The nurse needs to familiarize him/herself with the person's street life due to misinterpretation of unusual behaviors.

   b. The homeless person is likely to be untrustworthy and may not provide accurate data.

   c. The homeless person is often psychotic and cannot relate to the nurse.

   d. The nurse needs to spend more time in the homeless person's environment, even being on the street with the person, so he/she can more easily make judgments about the person's values and belief systems.

10. What is the most dangerous aspect of providing antipsychotic medications to a homeless person?

    a. The person may sell the drugs to anyone on the street, and the drugs may have serious side effects.

    b. The homeless person may become drowsy and thus be placed in dangerous situations on the street.

    c. The homeless person is usually not able to find a safe storage container for medications.

    d. The homeless person often becomes more psychotic after being placed on antipsychotics, because they are unreliable in taking the required doses.

CHAPTER 12

Psychopharmacology

The development of psychopharmacology has paralleled the increasingly important role of the nurse in medication management. The administration of psychotropic medication involves specific nursing responsibilities. Specific client populations who may require psychotropic medication include pregnant and lactating women, older adults, and children and adolescents. Nurses must be aware of the specific management issues inherent in polypharmacy in clients' use of alternative substances to treat mental health disorders. Nurses can blend an understanding of psychosocial needs with specific symptoms to provide optimal nursing care. Nurses must engage in a research process that evaluates the multiple effects of medication on a client's life and functioning.

LEARNING OBJECTIVES

After completing the exercises in this workbook, and studying the corresponding chapter in the textbook, the student will be able to:

- Describe principles of psychopharmacology and why they are so important to the course of a client's treatment.

- Identify important classes and subclasses of psychotherapeutic drugs and the disorders for which they are commonly used.

- List the actions, mechanisms of action, therapeutic dosages, uses, side effects, potential toxicity, administration, contraindications, and nursing implications of various psychotropic medications.

- Explain how developments in psychopharmacology have changed the provision of and settings for psychiatric health care.

- Describe important components of the nursing process as they relate to medication management.

- Formulate a nursing care plan for a client whose treatment involves the use of psychotropic medication.

KEY TERMS

Adherence: A client's willingness to receive recommended drug treatment as prescribed by a caregiver.

Affinity: A drug's tendency to be found at a given receptor site.

Agonist: A drug that initiates a therapeutic effect by binding to a receptor.

Antagonist: A drug that binds to receptors without causing any regulatory effect; its action is to block the binding of an endogenous agonist.

Efficacy: The information encoded in a drug's chemical structure that causes the receptor to change accordingly when the drug is bound.

Loss of efficacy: The loss of ability to achieve a drug's maximum benefit.

Maximal efficacy: The maximal effect a drug can produce.

Neuroleptic malignant syndrome: A serious and potentially fatal side effect that accompanies the use of certain antipsychotic agents. Characteristics include severe muscular rigidity, altered consciousness, stupor, catatonia, hyperpyrexia, and labile pulse and blood pressure.

Polypharmacy: Use of two or more psychotropic drugs, two or more drugs of the same chemical class, or two or more drugs with the same or similar pharmacologic actions to treat different conditions.

Potency: The concentration of a drug in plasma.

Psychopharmacology: The study of the chemistry, disposition, actions, and clinical pharmacology of drugs used to treat psychiatric disorders.

Refractoriness: A state of desensitization in which a drug's effect diminishes with repeated or subsequent use of the same concentration.

Refractory mania: Bipolar disorder with mania that is completely unresponsive or marginally responsive to drug therapy with conventional mood-stabilizing agents.

Side effects: Dysfunctions and discomforts that a client experiences directly as a result of taking a medication.

Tardive dyskinesia: The most serious side effect of long-term use of neuroleptics, with often irreversible and severely disabling symptoms that include involuntary choreoathetotic movements affecting the face, tongue, and perioral, buccal, and masticatory muscles.

Target symptoms: The specific symptoms that a medication aims to change.

Chapter Outline

KEY TOPICS

Principles of psychopharmacotherapeutics: Agonists/antagonists, affinity, potency, efficacy, target symptoms, polypharmacy

Important psychotherapeutic drugs: Antidepressants, mood stabilizers, anxiolytics, antipsychotics, stimulants

Nursing care of the client receiving psychopharmacologic agents: Nursing process; special issues, such as pregnancy, children and adolescents, and older adults.

■ Exercises

MATCHING

Match the term in Part A with the statement that applies to the term in Part B.

PART A

a. affinity

b. agonist

c. potency

d. neuroleptic malignant syndrome

e. polypharmacy

f. antagonist

g. refractoriness

h. refractory mania

i. tardive dyskinesia

j. target symptoms

PART B

1. _____ A desensitization state in which a drug's effect diminishes with repeated use of the same concentration

2. _____ Serious and potentially fatal side effect characterized by muscular rigidity, stupor, and labile vital signs

3. _____ Symptoms that a medication aims to change

4. _____ Drug's tendency to be found at a given receptor site

5. _____ Completely unresponsive or marginally responsive to drug therapy with conventional mood-stabilizing agents

6. _____ Drug that initiates a therapeutic effect by binding to a receptor

7. _____ A serious side effect of chronic neuroleptic use characterized by involuntary movements and disabling symptoms

8. _____ Using two or more psychotropic drugs

9. _____ Concentration of drug in plasma

10. _____ Binds to a receptor without causing any regulatory effect

CREATE YOUR OWN PSYCHOPHARMACOLOGY STUDY GUIDE

Within your textbook chapter, you will find tables for each drug category that include usual dose, sedation level/half-life, side effects, and relief of symptoms. Using the textbook tables, fill in the blanks for each category of psychotropic medication on the accompanying chart (Table 12-1, Study Guide for Psychotropic Medications). Focus on nursing interventions that would be optimal for assisting the client taking the specified category of medication, and also major teaching points.

CRITICAL THINKING AND SELF-EVALUATION EXERCISES

1. If you were depressed, would you seek treatment? If a medication were suggested, would you take it? Why or why not?

2. Do you have a friend or relative who is on a psychotropic medication? If so, describe your response and thoughts about this when you found out.

3. Do you have any biases or stereotypes about people who are on psychotropic medications? If so, list these and think about why you feel this way. Examine whether or not these perceptions are changeable.

■ NCLEX-Style Exam Questions

1. Target symptoms for antidepressant medications include all except which of the following?
   a. Anhedonia
   b. Euthymic mood
   c. Change in appetite and sleep patterns
   d. Difficulty concentrating

2. Antidepressants are considered the treatment of choice for major depression; however, they should be used most cautiously in clients with a history of
   a. asthma and respiratory diseases.
   b. smoking.
   c. cardiac or seizure disorders.
   d. liver disease.

3. Laura, age 40, has bipolar disorder and has just begun a regimen of lithium, 600 mg tid. The most critical management issue for Laura during the first 2 weeks of treatment is
   a. ascertaining that she is taking a full dose daily.
   b. ensuring her blood levels reach a therapeutic and safe dose.
   c. educating her about the side effects of lithium.
   d. monitoring her cardiac status.

4. When Laura comes to the hospital for her 2-week follow-up, she complains of a hand tremor that keeps her from holding her coffee cup, feeling confused, stomach aches, and occasional tripping. The most therapeutic intervention of the psychiatric nurse would be to
   a. explain to Laura that these are common side effects and that they will subside soon.
   b. tell Laura that you and she will monitor these side effects to be sure they do not increase in severity.
   c. call Laura's psychiatrist, because her symptoms are indicative of moderate toxicity.
   d. ask Laura to return 3 days later to see the psychiatrist, who will be in the clinic on that day.

TABLE 12–1 Study Guide for Psychotropic Medications

Psychotropic Category	Nursing Interventions for the Individual Client	Critical Teaching Points for the Client and Family
Antidepressant: TCA and tetracyclics		
Antidepressant: MAOI's		
Antidepressant: SSRI's, SRI's		
Mood stabilizer: Lithium		
Mood stabilizer: Carbamazepine & divalproex		
Mood stabilizer: gabapentin, lamotrigine, primidone, pramipexol, nimodipine		
Anxiolytics: Buspar		
Anxiolytics: Benzodiazepines		
Antipsychotics: Typical high potency		
Antipsychotics: Typical low potency		
Antipsychotics: Atypical		

ADDITIONAL NOTES:

5. The lithium level that you might expect to see in Laura's case, considering her symptoms, is
   a. 0.04–0.05 mEq/L.
   b. 0.06–1.2 mEq/L.
   c. 1.5–2.0 mEq/L.
   d. 2.0–2.6 mEq/L.

6. Benzodiazepines work by the following mechanism of action:
   a. They act directly on dopaminergic neurons in the medulla.
   b. They act directly on GABA receptors and are thought to increase the amount of GABA available.
   c. They act indirectly through a second messenger to affect levels of circulating GABA.
   d. The mechanism of action of this category of drugs is unknown at this time.

7. The difference between traditional and atypical antipsychotics is that
   a. traditional antipsychotics work mostly as dopamine agonists, but antipsychotics work through antagonizing the dopamine receptor.
   b. traditional antipsychotics have a more powerful effect on the negative symptoms of schizophrenia, whereas atypical antipsychotics exert stronger effects on the positive symptoms.
   c. atypical antipsychotics work on dopamine-receptor and serotonin-receptor blockade, whereas traditional antipsychotics work on dopamine-receptor blockade.
   d. there are no major differences between these two classes of drugs; their advantages are that there is a wider spectrum of drugs from which to choose.

8. When working with a client who is being placed on psychotropic medications, all but which of

the following are important in assisting the client to adhere to his or her medical regimen?
   a. Keep in close contact, with careful follow-up.
   b. Listen to the client's complaints of side effects but do not jump to intervene because early complaints have been found to be based on fear more than the client's true experience with side effects.
   c. Develop a strong therapeutic alliance with the client, including frequent sessions and close monitoring.
   d. Understand and utilize the community and family supports that may be available to the client.

9. In regard to the principles of psychotropic medication management and administration with children and adolescent clients,
   a. the principles are the same for both.
   b. the principles differ significantly, including the importance of educating about side effects in children.
   c. the principles were developed in different decades, and so they do differ on some fine points.
   d. Psychotropics are rarely if ever prescribed for children.

10. When caring for an older adult on psychotropic medication, the psychiatric nurse must be aware that older adults
   a. are often refractory to psychotropic medications.
   b. are always reluctant to take these medications because of stigma and stereotyping.
   c. usually require a lower dose of these medications than do younger counterparts.
   d. are not as sensitive to the effects of the psychotropics, and so are usually given slightly higher doses than in younger people.

Spirituality in Psychiatric Care

Chapter 13 discusses spirituality, which has been described as a person's experience of, or a belief in, a power apart from his or her own existence. It also has been described as an individual search for meaning. There has been a resurgence of interest in spiritual and religious matters, and research has been conducted to document their beneficial effects on people's health. Various reasons are given for this resurgence, including the health benefits of a spiritual life, acknowledgment of the limits of medical care, discoveries in physics, and research in religion and mental health. It is crucial for nurses and other healthcare providers to become aware of their own personal values, their client's values, and the differences between both. This will help them to act from their own perspectives without imposing their values on others. The role of the nurse with respect to spirituality and religion is fraught with ethical concerns. Nurses can conduct a brief spiritual assessment, but in the absence of special training spiritual interventions are best implemented with the aid of clergy or spiritual healers of the client's choice.

LEARNING OBJECTIVES

After completing the exercises in this workbook, and studying the corresponding chapter in the textbook, the student will be able to:

- Discuss the concepts of spirituality and religion.

- Analyze the strengths and weaknesses of the research findings related to spirituality, religion, and mental health.

- Describe how religious and spiritual themes may be manifested in mental illnesses.

- Explore reasons for the resurgence of interest in the spiritual aspects of health care.

- Debate the importance of clarifying values and becoming self-aware in relation to implementing spiritual and religious interventions.

- Examine the role of clergy in mental health care.

- Discuss the components of spiritual assessment.

- List several spiritual coping practices and interventions the nurse might use when working with clients.

- Evaluate the importance of keeping ethical concerns in mind while attending to a client's spiritual and religious needs.

KEY TERMS

Bibliotherapy: The use of literature to help clients gain insight into feelings and behavior and learn new ways to cope with difficult situations.

Contemplation and meditation: Types of mental exercises that involve calmly limiting thought and attention.

Prayer: A kind of communication or conversation with a power that a person recognizes as divine.

Religion: The outward practice of a spiritual system of beliefs, values, codes of conduct, and rituals.

Rituals: Ceremonies, rites, or acts such as prayer, singing hymns, abstaining from food, water, or sexual relations, and using sacred emblems.

Spirituality: A person's experience of, or a belief in, a power apart from his or her own existence; an individual search for meaning.

Values: Ideals or beliefs that are important to people and that in large part determine how they act and behave.

Worship: The devotion accorded to a higher power or deity.

Chapter Outline

SPIRITUALITY AND RELIGION

SPIRITUALITY, RELIGION, AND MENTAL HEALTH AND ILLNESS
Illness Prevention
Spirituality, Religion, and Mental Illness
RELIGIOUS AND SPIRITUAL INTERVENTIONS IN MENTAL HEALTH CARE
Changing Attitudes and Philosophies
Clarifying Values
The Role of Clergy in Mental Health Care
The Role of the Nurse in Mental Health Care
Spiritual Assessment
Spiritual Coping Practices and Interventions
Prayer
Bibliotherapy with Sacred Writings

Contemplation and Meditation
Repentance and Forgiveness
Worship and Rituals
Fellowship and Altruistic Service
Journal Writing
ETHICAL CONCERNS

KEY TOPICS

Spirituality and religion: Relation to mental health and illness; illness prevention

Religious and spiritual interventions in mental health care: Attitudes, philosophies, values; role of clergy in mental health care; psychiatric nursing role including spiritual assessment, and spiritual coping practices and interventions

■ Exercises

SENTENCE COMPLETION

For the following, complete the sentences by filling in the blanks.

1. _____ has been described as an individual's search for meaning in life.

2. _____ seems to provide clients with social support as well as an effective cognitive schema that enhances well-being and lowers distress.

3. _____ care and _____ care have been linked throughout history, with healing being associated with appeasement of spirits or gods.

4. _____ are ideals or beliefs that are important to people and that often determine how they behave and act.

5. Many clients consider their _____ to be their primary mental health care provider.

CORRECT THE FALSE STATEMENTS

For the following, mark T for true or F for false, and correct those that are false.

1. _____ NANDA has identified specific nursing interventions for clients who are experiencing spiritual distress.

2. _____ A spiritual history is not appropriate for every client.

3. _____ Religious interventions are more often structured, denominational, external, cognitive, ritualistic, and public.

4. _____ Bibliotherapy, contemplation, and meditation are types of treatments that involve calmly limiting thought and attention.

5. _____ Devout nurses may see their work as a religious calling; therefore, there is not a moral objection to teaching, preaching, or otherwise attempting to assist clients to see that point of view.

CASE STUDY

Sharon was admitted to the inpatient unit with an acute schizophrenic episode. She is psychotic and speaks often of "God's wrath coming down on me," "my inner spirit has been crushed by the demons from hell," and "we are all at risk for the fires of hell." She asks frequently to speak with the hospital chaplain. Upon assessment, you find that Sharon is the daughter of a conservative Baptist preacher and prior to her illness had been very active in the church, including teaching Sunday school. She is planning to attend Bible Baptist College in the upcoming fall. Sharon has been placed on an antipsychotic medication. When she is stable and no longer psychotic, you begin to conduct a formal assessment of her spiritual status.

1. Develop a care plan for Sharon, considering the following:
   a. Assessment: What additional information will you gather when conducting a spiritual assessment of Sharon? List a nursing diagnosis.
   b. Planning: Establish one goal for Sharon around the spiritual diagnosis. How would you go about developing a spiritually appropriate plan of care for Sharon?
   c. Intervention: What are interventions that may be useful when working with Sharon on spiritual issues?
   d. Evaluation: How will you measure whether or not your interventions with Sharon have been successful?

CRITICAL THINKING AND SELF-EVALUATION EXERCISES

1. Do you practice spirituality or belong to a specific religion?

2. How does your spirituality influence your everyday behaviors and your ideas about nursing?

3. What would be your most difficult challenge if caring for a client who has dramatically different spiritual beliefs than yours? How might you deal with this?

■ NCLEX-Style Exam Questions

1. Which of the following would be *least* helpful in a spiritual assessment of a client who is seriously ill?
   a. "Is faith (religion, spirituality) important to you in this illness?"
   b. "Do you have someone to talk with about religious matters?"
   c. "How did you practice religion or spirituality when you were growing up?"
   d. "Would you like to explore religious matters with someone?"

2. Spiritual interventions are contraindicated in all except which of the following situations?
   a. The client is psychotic or delusional.
   b. The client is unwilling to participate.
   c. The client is a minor, and the parents are unaware that the child is participating.
   d. The client is taking high-dose phenothiazines, which create drowsiness and decreased concentration.

3. The psychiatrist who has been working with a client on his spirituality asks the client to read her book, "The Power of Spirituality on Thinking and Life," and to discuss it with her the following week. This is a form of:
   a. coercive therapy.
   b. contemplative therapy.
   c. transference.
   d. bibliotherapy.

4. The difference between worship and rituals is that worship denotes:
   a. partaking of sacraments.
   b. devotion that one gives to a higher power or deity.
   c. a ceremony that shows commitment.
   d. an act of prayer or song.

5. Spirituality and religion differ along the following lines:
   a. spirituality is a person's experience of, or belief in, a power apart from himself or herself, whereas religion is the outward practice of a spiritual system of beliefs.
   b. spirituality is the belief that one's spirit will go to Heaven or Hell upon death; religion is a way to ensure that the individual will go to Heaven.
   c. religion has been recognized for at least 3,000 years, whereas spirituality has been recognized for only 1,000–1,500 years.
   d. religion is more often used in clinical practice because it is easier to implement within an acute hospital setting than is spirituality.

6. All except which of the following are ways in which religion may assist the mentally ill client in illness prevention?
   a. Providing a support network for the client
   b. Providing a cognitive schema that can put symptoms and illness into perspective
   c. Providing strong support for taking psychotropic medications that the client desperately needs
   d. Providing guiding principles for life, including social and health-enhancing behaviors.

7. Spiritual and health care have been linked throughout history. Which of the following is a description of a way in which this has been evidenced?
   a. Healing is often linked to appeasing spirits or gods, or equilibration of an imbalanced life force.
   b. Establishment of psychiatric hospitals
   c. Training of mental health practitioners in both spiritual and health issues in psychiatry
   d. Clients often seeking out their health care providers for spiritual guidance.

8. Mrs. Clancy has been admitted with depression and has asked to speak with the hospital chaplain. What is your most therapeutic nursing intervention?

   a. "Mrs. Clancy, I will try my best to have the chaplain visit you as soon as possible."

   b. "Mrs. Clancy, because you are in the midst of your depression, it is best that you wait until symptoms resolve."

   c. "I would be more than happy to do so, but I'll need to speak with your family prior to calling the chaplain."

   d. "I realize this is important to you, Mrs. Clancy; however, it is more difficult to resolve your symptoms when religious issues are brought to the forefront."

9. Your client, Jonas, hints that he would like to discuss his spiritual and religious beliefs with someone. What is the best nursing intervention at this point?

   a. Speak with Jonas further about his needs to assess how best to intervene.

   b. Begin meeting with Jonas as often as he likes to discuss spirituality.

   c. Ask Jonas if he would like to speak with you on a daily basis; you pray daily and would be happy to include Jonas in your prayer sessions.

   d. Tell Jonas that you would like to speak with his wife regarding her perception of his spirituality and religious needs.

10. Chad, age 22, is admitted in a psychotic episode. His frequent requests to speak with the hospital chaplain are interspersed with profanities regarding God and the devil. Your most therapeutic nursing intervention would be to

    a. continue providing safe, effective care and give antipsychotic medications as ordered to reduce Chad's symptoms of psychosis.

    b. immediately call the chaplain, because you realize Chad's symptoms may resolve with spiritual counseling.

    c. call the chaplain and ask to meet with her and Chad when she comes to your unit so you can monitor the exchange.

    d. tell Chad you are not allowed to call the chaplain when he is this disturbed.

CHAPTER 14

Complementary and Alternative Medicine

Complementary and alternative healthcare and medical practice (CAM) refers to practices that are not considered conventional in Western medical practice. These practices are used instead of (alternative) or in addition to (complementary) mainstream medical practices. The ethical and legal considerations for CAM are manifold. Many considerations are related to federal regulation of herbal therapy, and client and primary health care provider collaboration on the use of herbal therapies. Legal considerations include required education or training with designated actions for licensure or certification for CAM therapies. Alternative systems of medical practice include traditional Chinese medicine, acupuncture, ayurvedic medicine, homeopathy, and naturopathy. Nurses have the opportunity to obtain information from the client, relate information to the client, and help blend CAM and traditional healing modalities. In addition, nurses can become intuitively adept at interacting and communicating with the energy system in the body.

LEARNING OBJECTIVES

After completing the exercises in this workbook, and studying the corresponding chapter in the textbook, the student will be able to:

- Define complementary and alternative medicine (CAM).

- Describe the current state of research of CAM therapies for psychiatric–mental health care.

- Discuss legal and ethical considerations for CAM.

- List the domains of CAM therapy.

- Provide examples of therapies within each domain.

- Understand the nurse's role in CAM therapy.

KEY TERMS

Aromatherapy: The use of essential oils to treat symptoms for physiological and psychological benefits.

Healing touch/Therapeutic touch: Two methods of "energy healing" that incorporate the therapist's intention to heal through either actual touch or non-touch repatterning of energy fields around the person.

Licensure: A mandatory process through which a government agency regulates a profession.

Mantras: Sounds, short words, or phrases repeated in the mind.

Meditation: A state of consciousness and an experience of the mind in which one tries to achieve awareness without thought.

Naturopathy: A range of therapies referred to as *natural medicine*; a way of life in which the body innately knows how to maintain health and heal itself.

Professional certification: A voluntary process that grants recognition to people for having met certain qualifications.

Ta'i chi: A Chinese blend of exercise and energy work with a series of choreographed, continuous slow movements performed with mental concentration and coordinated breathing.

Yoga: A manipulative, body-based method that teaches basic principles of spiritual, mental, and physical energies to promote health and wellness.

Chapter Outline

OVERVIEW OF COMPLEMENTARY AND ALTERNATIVE MEDICINE
National Center for Complementary and Alternative Medicine and CAM Expansion
Prevalence of Complementary and Alternative Medicine
Research Studies
Ethical and Legal Considerations
CLASSIFICATION OF COMPLEMENTARY AND ALTERNATIVE MEDICINE
Alternative Systems of Medical Practice
Traditional Chinese Medicine (TCM)
Acupuncture
Ayurvedic Medicine

Naturopathy
Homeopathy
Mind–body Interventions
Meditation
Imagery
Music Therapy
Spiritual Healing and Prayer
Biological-Based Therapies
Herbal Therapies
Aromatherapy
Manipulative and Body-Based Methods
T'ai Chi
Yoga
Massage
Energy Therapies
Biofield Therapies
Healing Touch and Therapeutic Touch
Reiki
Bioelectromagnetic-Based Therapies
THE NURSE'S ROLE

KEY TOPICS

Complementary and alternative medicine: Prevalence, research, ethical and legal considerations

Classification of complementary and alternative medicine: Alternative systems of medical practice; mind–body interventions; biological-based therapies, manipulative and body-based therapies, energy therapies

The nurse's role in complementary and alternative medicine

■ Exercises

MATCHING

Match the domain of CAM therapy in Part A with the type of intervention that is included in that category. You may use domain numbers multiple times.

PART A

a. alternative systems of practice

b. mind–body interventions

c. biological-based therapies

d. manipulative and body-based methods

e. energy therapies

PART B

1. _____ Acupuncture

2. _____ Yoga

3. _____ Healing touch

4. _____ Ayurvedic medicine

5. _____ Massage

6. _____ Reiki

7. _____ Meditation

8. _____ T'ai chi

9. _____ Homeopathy

10. _____ Aromatherapy

11. _____ Naturopathy

12. _____ Biofield therapies

13. _____ Magnetic therapy

14. _____ Imagery

15. _____ Herbal therapy

16. _____ Music therapy

17. _____ Therapeutic touch

18. _____ Hydrotherapy

SHORT ANSWER

1. List five basic principles underlying CAM, as identified by Eliopoulos.

   _____

   _____

   _____

   _____

2. Give three purposes for the National Center for Complementary and Alternative Medicine (NCCAM).

   _____

   _____

   _____

3. All CAM therapies are divided into five domains. List these domains, and give examples of practices in each.

   _____

   _____

   _____

   _____

4. List five benefits of acupuncture.

_____

_____

_____

_____

■ NCLEX-Style Exam Questions

1. Complementary medicine is best defined as
   a. medicine that helps the client to enhance self-esteem.
   b. unconventional medical practices that are used in combination with typical medical care.
   c. medicines that are integrated routinely into medical school training and yet are not used widely.
   d. techniques used by nurses and case managers but very rarely by physicians.

2. Complementary medicine is often also called
   a. alternative.
   b. unconventional.
   c. integrative.
   d. atypical.

3. The NCCAM was established in 1992. By 2002, it
   a. has had a decline in interest and funding that has contributed to the non-use of these types of interventions by traditional health care providers.
   b. has experienced a rebirth because of consumers' dissatisfaction with increased costs, managed care, and lack of personal interactions with their medical care providers.
   c. has not regrouped since the stock market crash.
   d. has focused on the training of traditional medical care providers in alternative and complementary interventions, particularly herbal remedies.

4. In 1997, the number of adults between the age of 35 and 49 years who were using at least one method of CAM was
   a. 4%.
   b. 50%.
   c. 15%.
   d. 90%.

5. Ethical issues around the use of CAM include all except which of the following?
   a. The FDA has no authority over herbal products.
   b. Very few botanicals sold in the United States have been tested in controlled clinical trials.
   c. Practitioners need to know about vitamins, herbs, or energy treatments and often are unaware that their clients use such treatments.
   d. Use of CAM by providers who are licensed as alternative but not complementary therapists.

6. Traditional Chinese medicine is based on the principle of
   a. internal balance and harmony.
   b. energy fields that regulate human states of being.
   c. meridians in the body that follow the circulatory system.
   d. the body knowing how to maintain health and to heal itself.

7. All except which of the following mind–body interventions are used in traditional, mainstream medical practice?
   a. Imagery
   b. Relaxation therapy
   c. Biofeedback
   d. Music therapy

8. Herbal therapy is:
   a. also called phytomedicine—using plants or plant parts to achieve therapeutic cures.
   b. a new technique that was begun by a physicians' group in California in 1991.
   c. not used often because of the dangers involved in overdose with many herbs
   d. a common form of therapy used in the Virgin Islands.

9. Yoga dates to 3000 B.C. and means "union" in Sanskrit. It is best characterized by which of the following?

  a. Slow exercise and blunt low force

  b. Choreographed, slow movements performed with coordinated breathing

  c. Using principles of spiritual, mental, and physical energies to promote health

  d. Manipulation of soft tissue in the body

10. Use of complementary modalities by nurses is most dependent on

  a. the nurse's individual state licensure board guidelines.

  b. the client signing an informed consent.

  c. the use of only herbal remedies.

  d. the nurse's prior training in a wide range of CAM.

CHAPTER 15

Community Mental Health, Support, and Rehabilitation

Community support is critical to the quality of life of individuals with severe mental illness who live in the community. The goal of community support systems is to enable those with severe mental illnesses to remain in the community while functioning at optimal levels of independence. A community support system encourages participation from all people within it: clients, family members, government officials, and providers. Essential components of a community support system include active outreach efforts, help in ensuring access to services, psychosocial and vocational opportunities, rehabilitative and supportive housing options, crisis intervention services, case management, and family and community education programs. Nurses serve as an important link between hospital and community and bring essential knowledge and skills to a community-based treatment team or a school IEP team. Nurses have a leadership role in the development of comprehensive systems committed to the holistic approach of intervening at both client and community levels.

LEARNING OBJECTIVES

After completing the exercises in this workbook, and studying the corresponding chapter in the textbook, the student will be able to:

- Identify the levels of prevention of mental illness.

- Describe potential interventions for primary, secondary, and tertiary prevention of mental health problems.

- Define the term "community support system."

- Describe the philosophical context of the community support initiative.

- Identify the essential components of a community support system.

- Compare at least five models for the delivery of community support services.

- Understand the development and functioning of systems of care for children who have multisystem needs and their families.

- Explain the relationship of case management/service coordination to the effectiveness of a community support system.

- Identify the trends that affect social policy regarding the care of persons with severe mental illnesses.

- Describe the nurse's role in community mental health care, using each step of the nursing process.

KEY TERMS

Aggregate group: A group identified as having at least one commonality among its members.

Aggregate mental health: The degree to which families and groups within a given environment contribute to, enhance, or intensify interaction among individuals along the mental health/illness continuum.

Case manager: A person who coordinates the various services that address the needs (e.g., housing, health care, mental health treatment, social contacts, workups) of a mentally ill client.

Community support system: A network of caring and responsible people committed to assisting a vulnerable population to meet its needs and develop its potential without becoming unnecessarily isolated or excluded from the community.

Primary prevention: Health care interventions designed to prevent mental disorders or to reduce identified mental disorders and disabilities within a population.

Secondary prevention: Health care interventions designed to identify mental health problems early and reduce their duration and prevalence.

Systems of care: Comprehensive spectrums of mental health and other necessary services organized into coordinated networks so that providers can more appropriately address the various and changing needs of children and adolescents with serious emotional disturbances and their families.

Tertiary prevention: Health care interventions designed to provide rehabilitation for clients with diagnosed disorders and to minimize the residual effects for people within a community who have mental health problems.

Chapter Outline

KEY TOPICS

Community mental health: History; primary, secondary, and tertiary prevention

Components of a community mental health system: Principles; models, including psychosocial rehabilitation model, Fairweather Lodge model, training in community living model, consumer-run alternative models, community worker models, community support programs, child and adolescent service system program

Public policy and trends: Chronicity of severe mental illness, stalled resources, poverty, reinstitutionalization, education, stigma, reforms

Nursing process in community settings

■ Exercises

MATCHING

Match the term in Part A with the statement that applies to the term in Part B.

PART A

a. case manager

b. psychosocial rehabilitation model

c. aggregate mental health

d. primary prevention

e. advance directive

f. secondary prevention

g. community support system

h. community mental health

i. tertiary prevention

j. aggregate group

PART B

1. _____ An example is a psychosocial club with members who fully participate in the program's operation.

2. _____ Self-help training group for clients with schizophrenia

3. _____ A document stating a consumer's intentions about choices of treatment prior to needing hospitalization for acute symptoms

4. _____ Teaching a high-school class about HIV+ disease

5. _____ Has at least one commonality among its members

6. _____ Focuses on collective mental health of all people in a community

7. _____ Degree to which families and groups in an environment contribute to interaction among individuals along the mental illness/health continuum

8. _____ Identifying relapse symptoms and teaching the client and family how to spot and manage them

9. _____ Coordinates various functions that address individual needs

10. _____ Network of people who are committed to assisting a vulnerable population to meet their needs

SHORT ANSWER

1. Briefly discuss some of the historical factors that have contributed to the development of community mental health. Include the prevailing philosophy of the time, and major events that pushed this movement forward.

2. Provide one example of an activity that you would find a community mental health nurse doing for each of the following levels of prevention: primary, secondary, and tertiary.

CASE STUDY

You are a community health nurse who has just been called for a referral to the local high school. The principal states that the school had a suicide a month ago, and in the last week a "very popular, totally happy, and wonderful young 15-year-old girl" took her life in an apparent overdose. The principal has asked you to address the mental health care needs of the students, grades 11 and 12. He has been deluged with students in his office and the office of the school psychologist. These students often come in groups; they are sad and emotional and cannot concentrate on their schoolwork. He is asking for support from the local community health nursing agency.

1. Assessment: What are the primary reasons for the principal's call? What data from this case study indicates that the referral is appropriate? List two diagnoses that are appropriate for this school system.

2. Planning: What are the students' most immediate needs. Provide at least one short-term and one long-term goal for each diagnosis.

3. Intervention: Discuss how you will intervene to meet the needs of this community. Is your intervention primary, secondary, or tertiary prevention?

4. Evaluation: Give several criteria by which you can determine if your interventions have been successful. Link the evaluation criteria to your diagnoses.

■ NCLEX-Style Exam Questions

1. Community mental health can be best described as
   a. treating the community as client.
   b. treating mentally ill individuals in a community program.
   c. treating the client by establishing community programs for his or her needs.
   d. treating the family as client, and considering both to be within a community.

2. The goal of the 1963 Community Health Centers Act was to
   a. provide treatment of the mentally ill within a community setting, not within hospitals.
   b. build health centers that were adjacent to mental institutions so that clients could still receive care but be independent.
   c. establish community living, vocational, and rehabilitation programs to assist individuals who were being deinstitutionalized.
   d. allow for the training and education of family members to assume care of their mentally ill members.

3. What was the original purpose for developing the role of the case manager in community-based care?
   a. To relieve already-burdened psychiatrists from having to make home visits to critically mentally ill clients
   b. To reduce stress on the emergency system (i.e. ambulances, 911 services), which were increasingly being taxed by mentally ill individuals and their families
   c. To allow the case manager to coordinate the various functions (housing, work-ups, social contacts, mental health treatment, etc.) that would address the needs of the mentally ill client within the community and reduce inpatient admissions
   d. To provide more comprehensive mental health psychotherapy to clients who were homebound

4. Susan, a case manager, is working with Mindy Jones, whose son Todd has schizophrenia. Mindy reports sadness, frequent crying, and fatigue. Susan works with her to establish some scheduling for rest, relaxation, and respite from caring for her son. At which level of prevention is Susan working with Mindy?
   a. Secondary
   b. Tertiary
   c. Primary
   d. Quarternary

5. Susan makes a home visit to the Jones household and finds that Todd has become psychotic in the prior 3 days and has bolted himself in his room. Susan works to encourage Todd to come out and calls the ambulance to take him to the emergency department. At what level of prevention is Susan working with Todd?
   a. Primary
   b. Secondary
   c. Tertiary
   d. Quarternary

6. All except which of the following are elements of a community support system?
   a. Identification of at-risk populations
   b. Adequate mental health care
   c. Provision of individual psychotherapy in the home if needed
   d. Case management responsible for helping the individual to make informed choices about care

7. Philosophical concepts behind community mental health care services include:
   a. Self-determination
   b. Normalization of settings as well as offerings
   c. Least restrictive appropriate settings
   d. Dependency needs must be met

8. A community mental health model program that incorporates membership responsibility in maintaining and advancing the program and social/recreational, vocational, residential, and educational services is called:
   a. psychosocial rehabilitation model.
   b. Fairweather Lodge model.
   c. community living model.
   d. community worker model.

9. Why has it been critical to design models of community mental health support for children and young people?
   a. Children and youths with emotional/behavioral difficulties, as a group, have the poorest long-term outcomes of any group with a disability.
   b. Children and young people have higher recidivism rates in prisons than any other group of inmates.
   c. Parents of these children give up and abandon them, leaving them vulnerable.
   d. Children and youths have unique needs that have never been addressed in psychiatry.

10. John, who was unemployed and mentally ill, was receiving an SSI check each month for 10 years. He was just trained in food services and has gotten a job at the local hamburger stop as a dishwasher. What is one disadvantage of John's getting a job?
   a. He will now become dependent on his place of employment to meet needs that were previously met in his psychosocial club.
   b. He now does not receive the health care benefit that he received as a full-time disabled person through SSI.
   c. He is now dependent on his job for a living.
   d. He will have to find a way to get shelter because he has lost his SSI-supported apartment.

CHAPTER 16

Behavioral Health Home Care

Home health care nursing and behavioral health home health care nursing are aspects of community health nursing and the community health movement. Behavioral health home health care attempts to assist the client and family to gain, regain, maintain, or restore the optimal state of health and independence; to minimize and rehabilitate the effects of illnesses and disability before or after institutionalization; and to prevent institutionalization altogether when possible. The nursing process is used by the behavioral health home health care nurse to provide comprehensive services to clients in their places of residence. Various social, legislative, and political forces make it likely that the need and demand for behavioral health home health care services will continue to increase.

LEARNING OBJECTIVES

After completing the exercises in this workbook, and studying the corresponding chapter in the textbook, the student will be able to:

- Describe the historical, philosophical, and theoretical foundations of behavioral health home care nursing practice.

- Identify the essential components of behavioral health home care nursing practice.

- Discuss appropriate candidates for behavioral health home care nursing services.

- Discuss ways that nurses modify the steps of the nursing process when caring for a client and family in the home.

KEY TERMS

Behavioral health clinical nurse specialist: A master's-prepared nurse with skills in psychiatric and mental health assessment and intervention who is eligible for, or has already received, ANA certification as a specialist in adult psychiatric and mental health nursing.

Home care: Part of a comprehensive health and mental health care system that aims to provide an array of health-related services to clients and families in their places of residence.

Chapter Outline

FOUNDATIONS OF BEHAVIORAL HEALTH HOME CARE
History of Behavioral Health Home Care
Principles of Behavioral Health Home Care
Home Care Services
Home Care Providers
Goals of Behavioral Health Home Care
BEHAVIORAL HEALTH HOME CARE NURSING
Behavioral Health Clinical Nurse Specialists
Attitudes and Feelings
The Nursing Process and Behavioral Health Home Care
Assessment
   Indicators and Standards of Care
   Data to Collect
   Data Gathering Methods
Nursing Diagnosis
Planning
Implementation
Evaluation
Trends in Behavioral Health Home Care Nursing

KEY TOPICS

Behavioral health home care: Principles, goals, services, and providers

Behavioral health home care nursing: Clinical nurse specialist, attitudes and feelings, and the nursing process in behavioral health home care

■ Exercises

MATCHING

Match the term in Part A with the statement that applies to the term in Part B.

PART A

a. home care
b. indications for need for behavioral health home care
c. social force influencing delivery of home health care nursing services
d. desired characteristics of behavioral health home care nurses
e. behavioral health clinical nurse specialist

PART B

1. _____ Has a master's degree in psychiatric and mental health; able to assess and intervene in the client's home

2. _____ Arranged to provide a variety of health-related services in the client's home

3. _____ Mental health status changes or impairment, multiple medical problems, family changes, motivation changes

4. _____ Good physical assessment skills and superb clinical judgment

5. _____ Percentage of older Americans is disproportionate to the total population.

SHORT ANSWER

1. What types of services are included under the umbrella of home health care services?

2. What are the goals of behavioral health home care?

3. What are critical indicators of the need for behavioral health home care?

4. Design three short-term and three long-term goals when working with a client in his or her home.

CORRECT THE FALSE STATEMENTS

For each of the following statements, correct the words that are underlined.

1. Home care has been delivered in the United States since the 1920s.

   _____

2. It was not until Medicare added "psychiatric" home care as a reimbursable service that nurses began to hold conferences around behavioral health care.

   _____

3. Two goals of home health care are to gain, regain, maintain, or restore the client's optimal state of health and independence and to minimize the symptoms clients experience while they are in the hospital.

   _____

4. A behavioral health clinical nurse specialist is a BSN-prepared nurse who has had specialized education for assessment and intervention skills and is ANA certified in psychiatric nursing.

   _____

5. In accordance with the *ANA Standards of Nursing*, the behavioral health home care nurse assesses the client and family.

   _____

CRITICAL THINKING AND SELF-EVALUATION EXERCISES

1. Have you ever had a family member receive home health care? If so, what was the greatest difficulty with the client that merited home health care?

2. Discuss your opinions about federal money (your tax dollars) going to support ill and disabled clients in their homes. Do you feel it is a good use of these dollars? How would you suggest the management of ill/disabled persons in a different way?

■ NCLEX-Style Exam Questions

1. All except which of the following describe behavioral health home care?

   a. A specialty service provided in the home

   b. Provides psychiatric and chemical dependency treatment, health teaching and wellness, and illness prevention

   c. Can be nontherapeutic and usually costs much more than an inpatient stay

   d. Is one part of a comprehensive health and mental health care system

2. What event triggered the process of supporting mental clients in society through deinstitutionalization and a focus on community care versus hospital-based care?

   a. The 1994 National Psychiatric Home Care Conference

   b. The 1979 addition by Medicare of "psychiatric" home care as a reimbursable service

   c. The 1983 report of the Joint Commission of Mental Illness and Health

   d. The establishment, in 1950, of the first home health care nursing service in Boston

3. All except which of the following are basic principles of behavioral health home care?

   a. The client is considered as an individual, treated separately and apart from his or her family unit.

   b. The whole individual must be considered.

   c. Cost-effective care requires direct payment at the level of program delivery.

   d. High-quality long-term care should be affordable.

4. What is the primary determinant of which services need to be arranged and coordinated in the home?

   a. The client's source of income

   b. The client's symptoms

   c. The individual needs of the client and family

   d. The overall needs of normal clients and families

5. All except which of the following are goals of behavioral health home care?

   a. Teaching problem-solving

   b. Providing respite

   c. Educating clients and their families

   d. Using a variety of techniques to control acute symptoms

6. Which is one of the most common population groups to be served through behavioral health home care?

   a. People over age 65

   b. People who are chronically suicidal

   c. People who are chronically psychotic

   d. People who are on multiple medication regimens

7. What is the recommended preparation for a behavioral health clinical nurse specialist?

   a. MS degree; ANA certified in adult psychiatric and mental health nursing

   b. AD degree with significant specialized training in psychiatric nursing; ANA certified as a psychiatric-mental health nurse

   c. BSN degree; within the past 5 years, at least 2 years of acute inpatient experience in psychiatry

   d. MSN degree with additional training in management of acute symptoms

8. The following statement would indicate that the behavioral health home care nurse has characteristics that impede her effectiveness in this role:

   a. "I am an organized person and never have difficulty finding documents."

   b. "I have worked in an acute inpatient psychiatric setting for 2 years and then worked in the Medical ICU the past year."

   c. "I sometimes feel unsafe in clients' homes, and carry my cell phone with me."

   d. "I have a difficult time with clients who have several different needs at the same time."

9. Which of the following is *not* a critical indicator of the need for behavioral health home care?

    a. Change in mental health status

    b. Inability to get transportation to health services

    c. Functional limitations

    d. Psychiatric crisis or emergency

10. Which is true of the nursing process in behavioral home health care?

    a. It is a joint process that includes the nurse and the client and his/her family.

    b. It is very different from the acute setting, because the nurse does not typically diagnose the client.

    c. Nursing interventions are not a large part of the behavioral home health care model, because many cannot realistically be done in a home setting.

    d. It is similar to that of the nursing process in other settings, with the exception that the family is the evaluator of whether or not care has been effective.

Violence and Abuse Within the Community

Chapter 17 discusses a topic that has emerged as critical within the past decade in the United States. Community violence is an umbrella term for numerous forms of aggression that individuals inflict on one another. It includes phenomena such as youth violence, intimate partner violence, child maltreatment, elder abuse, and rape and sexual assault. One way to understand community violence is to consider not just traits of the perpetrator but factors within the family, community, and culture that place individuals at risk for becoming a victim or perpetrator of violence. The tremendous increase in the incidence of youth violence has been explained by individual traits as well as family, school, community, and neighborhood influences.

Rape and sexual assault are acts of violence in the form of sexual behaviors that are forcefully perpetrated upon another, violating the victim's person and shattering his or her sense of safety and predictability in the world. Rape trauma syndrome details the sequence of psychological events rape victims may experience following an attack. The nursing care of the rape victim involves attending to both physical and psychological needs and requires particular sensitivity to the victim's reaction. To intervene with the rape victim effectively, nurses must attend to and control their own reaction to the event.

LEARNING OBJECTIVES

After completing the exercises in this workbook, and studying the corresponding chapter in the textbook, the student will be able to:

- Understand the scope and sources of community violence.

- Describe a model that organizes the multiple conditions that support the phenomenon of community violence.

- Explain the key factors that place a youth at risk for developing violent responses to life situations.

- Identify the dynamics of intimate partner violence and the nurse's role in recognizing, screening, and assisting its victims.

- Discuss the effects of maltreatment on a child's development.

- Identify the scope of elder abuse and key prevention strategies.

- Define rape and sexual assault.

- Describe the phases of the rape trauma syndrome and treatment approaches.

- Apply the nursing process to the care of the trauma survivor.

- Understand the importance of clarifying one's attitudes before intervening with rape victims.

KEY TERMS

Ecological model: A perspective that holds that certain behaviors result from the interaction of individuals' traits with contextual factors arising from the family, community, and culture in which they reside.

Elder abuse: Mistreatment of older adults, which includes physical abuse, physical neglect, sexual abuse, psychological abuse or neglect, financial abuse, and violation of personal rights.

Intimate partner violence: Violence occurring between persons (same or opposite sex) who have a current or former relationship (i.e., dating, marital, or cohabiting). Violent acts include both physical and sexual violence as well as threats and psychological/emotional abuse.

Maltreatment: Behavior toward another person that is outside the norms of conduct and involves a significant risk of causing physical or emotional harm; four categories are recognized: physical abuse, sexual abuse, neglect, and emotional maltreatment.

Public health approach: A method of addressing social problems that holds that multiple causes must be met with solutions that address each level of the problem.

Rape: A crime of forced or coerced sexual penetration (oral, anal, or vaginal) of a nonconsenting person.

Sexual assault: Forced or coerced sexual acts performed on a nonconsenting person.

Statutory rape: Rape of a minor.

Violence: The threatened or actual use of physical force by an individual that results or has a high likelihood of resulting in psychological or physical injury or death.

Chapter Outline

THE ECOLOGICAL MODEL OF VIOLENCE
Macrosystem
Microsystem
Exosystem
Ontogenic Development
PUBLIC HEALTH APPROACH TO VIOLENCE PREVENTION
YOUTH VIOLENCE
Risk and Protective Factors for Youth Violence
Individual Risk Factors
Family Risk Factors
Peer Risk Factors
Neighborhood Risk Factors
Protective Factors
Public Health Approach to Youth Violence
Nurse's Role in Youth Violence Prevention Efforts
FAMILY VIOLENCE
Intimate Partner Violence
Defining the Scope of IPV
Cost to Children
Addressing Intimate Partner Violence
 Problems with Detection and Screening
 Importance of Screening
Nurse's Role in the Identification and Treatment of IPV
Child Maltreatment
Effects of Maltreatment on Child Function
 Social Functioning
 Behavioral Functioning
 Emotional and Intellectual Functioning
 Health and Physical Functioning
 Family Functioning and Parenting Practices
Nurse's Role in the Identification of Maltreatment
Elder Abuse
Types
Causes
Nurse's Role in the Identification and Treatment of Elder Abuse
RAPE AND SEXUAL ASSAULT
Types of Rape
Rape by a Stranger
Date Rape and Acquaintance Rape
Marital Rape
Rape Trauma Syndrome
Additional Ramifications of Rape

Treatment for Survivors of Rape or Sexual Assault
Psychopharmacologic Interventions
Psychological Interventions
Rape Prevention
Nurses' Role in the Assessment and Treatment of Rape and Trauma Victims
Assessment
Treatment

KEY TOPICS

Ecological model of violence: Macrosystem, microsystem, exosystem

Youth violence: Risk and protective factors, public health approaches, nursing role

Family violence: Intimate partner violence, child maltreatment, elder abuse

Rape and sexual assault: Rape trauma syndrome, survivor treatment, rape prevention; nursing role in rape prevention

■ Exercises

MATCHING

Match the term in Part A with the statement that applies to the term in Part B.

PART A

a. child neglect

b. sexual assault

c. public health approach to violence

d. microsystem

e. maltreatment

f. intimate partner violence

g. physical abuse

h. ecological model

i. rape

j. rape trauma syndrome

PART B

1. _____ Violence occurring between two persons who have a current or former relationship

2. _____ Forced or coerced sexual acts performed on a nonconsenting person

3. _____ Examples are scalding, beatings with an object, severe physical punishment.

4. _____ Behavior toward another person that is outside norms and involves risk of causing serious emotional or physical harm

5. _____ Holds that multiple causes of violence must be met with multilevel solutions

6. _____ Perspective that certain behaviors result from individuals' traits with contextual factors from the family, community, and culture in which they reside

7. _____ Examples are leaving a child unattended and keeping him or her out of school.

8. _____ Characterized by disorganization, integration, and resolution of the experience

9. _____ Includes formal and informal structures that make up children's and their family's world

10. _____ A crime of forced or coerced sexual penetration of a nonconsenting person

SHORT ANSWER

1. List at least three of each of the following factors that contribute to the epidemic of youth violence in our country: individual risk factors, family risk factors, peer risk factors, and neighborhood risk factors.

2. Define intimate partner violence. Discuss uniform definitions that are being developed and how IPV affects children.

3. What might be the most significant factor or barrier in detecting and intervening in IPV?

4. Why is screening so important in IVP?

5. List the effects of maltreatment on a child's social functioning, behavioral functioning, emotional and intellectual functioning, and health and physical functioning.

CRITICAL THINKING AND SELF-EVALUATION EXERCISES

1. Think about your own feelings about abuse of children and the elderly. What are your primary feelings? Describe why these feelings are elicited.

2. Evaluate your own feelings and biases around the issues of child abuse and neglect. Consider what your role will be as an RN if you encounter individuals who have experienced abuse of some

type. What might be the major obstacles to you in providing appropriate screening and referral? How might you overcome these obstacles?

■ NCLEX-Style Exam Questions

1. All except which of the following are indicators of physical abuse of an elder?
   a. Intimidation of the elderly person
   b. Bruises
   c. Frequent ER visits with unexplained trauma
   d. Dislocations or sprains

2. Mrs. Jacobs has been attending a local day program. Her counselor there notices that she has been coming in with bruises and scrapes and is increasingly depressed. On physical examination, Mrs. Jacobs is diagnosed with genital herpes. Which type of elder abuse do you suspect?
   a. Physical neglect
   b. Sexual abuse
   c. Psychological abuse
   d. Financial abuse

3. All except the following are considered risk factors for being a victim of elder abuse?
   a. Over 65 years of age
   b. Female
   c. Impaired cognitive function
   d. Financial dependency

4. Rape trauma syndrome is a two-phase process that all rape survivors experience. It includes
   a. an acute phase of disorganization and a long-term process of reorganization.
   b. an acute phase of symptom exaggeration and a short-term phase of reintegration.
   c. a phase of psychosis followed by a phase of recovery.
   d. exacerbation of symptoms, and a successful recovery phase.

5. The following are frequently experienced during the first phase of rape trauma syndrome:
   a. fear, anxiety, disbelief, anger, and shock.
   b. fear, depression, anxiety, anger, and withdrawal.
   c. depression, anxiety, resolution, and mental comfort.

d. resolving feelings, seeking support, crying, and difficulty sleeping.

6. If recovery from the rape does not occur, the victim may develop:
   a. anxiety disorders.
   b. post-traumatic distress syndrome.
   c. borderline personality disorder
   d. delirium.

7. Which antidepressant has been the most helpful to victims of rape in managing symptoms through recovery?
   a. SSRIs
   b. MAOIs
   c. TCAs
   d. Olanzapine

8. According to Herman, the treatment of individuals who have been traumatized has three stages:
   a. safety; remembrance and mourning; and reconnection.

b. connection, working through, and resolution.
c. consolation, bereavement, and rebirth.
d. Rebirth, resolution, and consolidation of self.

9. A college program aimed at teaching female students about ways to keep themselves safe from attack or rape while walking on campus would be considered:
   a. primary prevention.
   b. secondary prevention.
   c. tertiary prevention.
   d. quaternary prevention.

10. All except which of the following are protective factors for children who are abused?
    a. Solid intelligence
    b. Easy disposition
    c. Aggressiveness toward potential offenders
    d. Secure attachments

CHAPTER 18

The Client With an Anxiety Disorder

This chapter will focus on the anxiety disorders. Anxiety is a normal response to a threatening situation; however, prolonged anxiety in the absence of threat is abnormal. Anxiety disorders are the most frequently occurring of all psychiatric syndromes, affecting children, adolescents, adults, and older adults. These disorders are often misdiagnosed and undertreated, compounding the problems they cause. Anxiety disorders are more common in women than men.

Levels of anxiety range from mild to moderate, severe, and panic. The client may report symptoms of dread, apprehension, restlessness, and jitteriness. Physiologic signs of anxiety may include increased heart rate, blood pressure, and depth and rate of respirations, and perspiration.

Common phobic disorders include agoraphobia, social phobia, and specific phobia. A panic disorder is characterized by recurrent, unpredictable panic attacks. Generalized anxiety disorder is characterized by chronic anxiety that is so uncomfortable it interferes with daily life. A person with obsessive–compulsive disorder experiences recurrent obsessions (persistent thoughts, images, or impulses) and compulsions (ritualistic behaviors performed routinely). Post-traumatic stress disorder is the development of certain characteristic symptoms after exposure to a severe, extraordinary, traumatic life experience.

Nonpharmacologic methods used to treat anxiety disorders in clients include relaxation techniques, such as deep breathing and progressive muscle relaxation; covert rehearsal; positive coping statements; cognitive reframing; systematic desensitization; and problem-solving strategies. Antianxiety medications commonly used to treat anxiety disorders are selective serotonin reuptake inhibitors (SSRIs), benzodiazepines (BZDs), buspirone, beta blockers, and tricyclic antidepressants (TCAs).

Assessment reference points for nurses include knowing the definition of anxiety and being able to recognize the signs and symptoms of different anxiety levels. Important interventions nurses perform in the care of clients with anxiety disorders include assisting the client through an anxiety attack, helping clients identify sources of anxiety, reinforcing use of adaptive coping mechanisms, and teaching new coping mechanisms. The nurse bases evaluation of whether nursing care for a client with an anxiety disorder is effective on the client's report of his or her feelings and observed behavior changes.

LEARNING OBJECTIVES

After completing the exercises in this workbook, and studying the corresponding chapter in the textbook, the student will be able to:

- Define the term "anxiety."

- Explain what is meant by "anxiety disorder."

- Describe the incidence and prevalence of anxiety disorders.

- Discuss proposed etiologies for anxiety disorders.

- Identify symptoms of anxiety disorders.

- Explain the different types of anxiety disorders.

- Discuss treatments for anxiety disorders.

- Apply the nursing process to the care of clients with anxiety disorders.

KEY TERMS

Acute stress disorder: An anxiety disorder in which symptoms of post-traumatic stress disorder appear within 4 weeks of exposure to the trauma and usually last less than 3 months.

Agoraphobia: A marked fear of being alone or in a public place from which escape would be difficult or help would be unavailable in the event of becoming disabled.

Anxiety: A sense of psychological distress that may or may not have a focus; it is a state of apprehension that may represent a response to environmental stress or a physical disease state.

Anxiety disorder: A group of conditions in which the affected person experiences persistent anxiety that he or she cannot dismiss and that interferes with his or her daily activities.

Compulsions: Ritualistic behaviors that a person feels compelled to perform either in accord with a specific set of rules or in a routine manner.

Generalized anxiety disorder: An anxiety disorder characterized by chronic and excessive worry and anxiety more days than not for at least 6 months and involving many aspects of the person's life; the worry and anxiety cause such discomfort as to interfere with daily life and relationships.

Obsessions: Recurrent, intrusive, and persistent ideas, thoughts, images, or impulses.

Obsessive–compulsive disorder: An anxiety disorder marked by recurrent obsessions or compulsions that are time-consuming (taking more than 1 hour per day) or that cause significant impairment or distress.

Panic attack: A discrete period of intense apprehension or terror without any real accompanying danger, accompanied by at least 4 of 13 somatic or cognitive symptoms.

Panic disorder: An anxiety disorder marked by recurrent, unexpected panic attacks that cause the affected person to worry persistently about recurrences or complications from the attacks or to undergo behavioral changes in response to the attacks for at least 1 month.

Phobia: A persistent, irrational fear attached to an object or situation that objectively does not pose a significant danger.

Post-traumatic stress disorder: An anxiety disorder marked by the development of characteristic symptoms after exposure to a severe or extraordinary stressor (eg, natural disasters, accidental or intentional human-made disasters), in which there is actual or threatened death, serious injury, or maiming to the self or others; occurs only in response to a traumatic life experience.

Social phobia: An anxiety disorder characterized by a persistent, irrational fear of and compelling desire to avoid situations in which the person may be exposed to unfamiliar people or to the scrutiny of others; fear of behaving in a way that may prove humiliating or embarrassing.

Chapter Outline

ANXIETY
The Continuum of Anxiety
Effects on Sensation
Effects on Cognition
Effects on Verbal Ability
Normal Versus Abnormal Anxiety
ANXIETY DISORDERS

Etiology
Neurobiological Theories
Psychological Theories
Signs and Symptoms/Diagnostic Criteria
Generalized Anxiety Disorder
Phobic Disorders
　Agoraphobia
　Social Phobia
　Specific Phobia
Panic Attacks
Panic Disorder
Obsessive–Compulsive Disorder
Post-traumatic Stress Disorder
Acute Stress Disorder
Comorbidities and Dual Diagnoses
Implications and Prognoses
Interdisciplinary Goals and Treatment
Psychodynamic Therapies
　Basic Cognitive Therapy Techniques for Anxiety
　Systematic Desensitization and Exposure Treatment
　Relaxation Techniques and Breathing Retraining
Pharmacologic Treatment
　Selective Serotonin Reuptake Inhibitors
　Benzodiazepines
　Buspirone
　Beta Blockers
　Tricyclic Antidepressants
APPLICATION OF THE NURSING PROCESS TO THE CLIENT WITH AN ANXIETY DISORDER
Assessment
Nursing Diagnosis
Planning
Implementation
Alleviating Anxiety
　Initiating a Therapeutic Dialogue
　Countering Faulty Thinking
　Managing Hyperventilation
　Suggesting Lifestyle Changes
Teaching Adaptive Coping Strategies
　Teaching Relaxation
　Teaching Problem-Solving Skills
Evaluation

KEY TOPICS

Continuum of Anxiety: Sensation, cognition, and verbal ability; normal vs. abnormal anxiety

Anxiety Disorders: Etiology; signs and symptoms; implications and prognosis; interdisciplinary goals and treatment

Nursing Process: Assessment, diagnosis, planning, implementation (alleviating anxiety, initiating therapeutic dialogue, countering faulty thinking, managing hyperventilation, suggesting lifestyle changes); teaching coping techniques (relaxation, problem-solving skills); evaluation

■ Exercises

CASE STUDY EXERCISE

June D., age 35, is single and lives alone in her subsidized apartment. She receives Social Security Disability monthly due to her disabling anxiety disorder. June comes to the local outpatient mental health center weekly for therapy with a psychiatric advanced practice registered nurse. Today, June comes into her therapist's office complaining that it took her an hour to make the 15-minute trip to the office. While driving down the street, June kept looking in her rear-view mirror and thinking that she had hit someone with her car. She pulled over and stopped her car to go back and check the road behind her, which was empty. She reports this happening three times on the way to the clinic; each time with increasing levels of anxiety. She arrives in a state of panic, tearful, wringing her hands, shaking, and complaining of shortness of breath and palpitations.

1. List two possible approaches to June at this time, and give your rationale for each. One example is provided.

    a. Possible Response (example): *"June, you seem to be very anxious. Can you talk about how you are feeling right now?"*

    Rationale: *June is having an episode of extreme anxiety following difficulty on the way to her appointment. It can be helpful to encourage June to talk about how she is feeling at this time, which can provide venting as well as increased insight into her feelings.*

    b. Possible Response: _____

    _____

    _____

    _____

    Rationale: _____

    _____

    _____

    _____

    c. Possible Response: _____

    _____

    _____

    _____

    _____

    Rationale: _____

    _____

    _____

    _____

June talks about feeling very frightened and worried that she may have killed someone on the way to her appointment. She says, "I have been feeling worse lately. Yesterday I was going to the grocery store, and I kept going back to check my stove. I kept thinking I hadn't turned it off. It took me 45 minutes to get out the front door; I must have rechecked it about 40 times. While I was at the store, I could hardly buy any food because I kept thinking that I had left the stove burning. I tried to put it out of my mind, but the thought kept coming back. I mean, I really do know that it's stupid, but I can't help it. Then, when I got home, I started to get really anxious because it seemed that the food had bugs all over it, I mean germs, you know? I had to wash everything before I put it away. This is just so time-consuming, and I hate it when I'm feeling this nervous."

2. From the data presented thus far in the case study, list June's symptoms. Categorize the symptoms into the following groups: cognitive, affective, physiological, and behavioral.

3. Consider June's symptoms, and make a decision about which of the anxiety disorders she may be experiencing. Include a rationale or criteria for making your choice. If there is more than one possibility, provide a summary of why you ruled the possibility in or out.

4. When assessing June's history and symptoms, list at least five clues you might look for that are often comorbid with anxiety disorders.

June's therapist is considering beginning a trial of fluvoxamine (Luvox), since June has never taken medications for her symptoms. Although June is hesitant about taking medications, she agrees to try and see if this medication will help her.

5. Which drug classification is fluvoxamine; how does fluvoxamine work at the level of the synapse, and what are the major side effects that the therapist will need to review with June?

6. What other medications might be considered for June's symptoms if the fluvoxamine does not work? List at least three other drugs in different classifications that could be used for June. Explain why you would or would not choose each of them.

7. How should the therapist begin this regimen? What effects might June experience as a result of the Luvox, especially within the first week of treatment, and how should the therapist prepare June for this?

June has been on the Luvox for about 2 weeks and reports that she is feeling less anxious in general. However, she comes to a session saying, "I keep having these feelings that I'm going to lose my apartment because I just can't keep it clean. I mean, I try to, but sometimes I am just so busy checking on things that I can't do my regular housekeeping."

8. If the therapist were to use a cognitive therapy approach with June during this session, discuss how she might address June's complaints. Provide three cognitive strategies that you could use with June to talk about her apartment.

9. Discuss at least one other strategy or technique that the therapist could use to work with June regarding her fears of losing her apartment.

June has been on the Luvox for about 6 weeks now and comes to her weekly therapy session stating, "I feel so much better! I'm not worried as much, and I'm not spending so much of my time checking everything. It is so great! I think I could concentrate enough to maybe get a very part-time job somewhere, but I'm not sure."

10. List at least two nursing diagnoses for June at this point. Complete the Nursing Process Worksheet on the next page for each of the diagnoses.

CRITICAL THINKING AND SELF-EVALUATION EXERCISES

1. Describe how you feel when you are mildly, moderately, and extremely anxious.

2. How does anxiety affect your concentration?

3. Discuss techniques you have used to deal with your own anxiety; share with your classmates.

■ NCLEX-Style Exam Questions

1. Susan has begun to wash her hands every hour on the hour because she fears that if germs become embedded in her skin, she will contract cancer. Which of the following would best describe Susan's behavior?
   a. An obsession
   b. A compulsion
   c. A panic attack
   d. Acute stress disorder

2. One major difference between post-traumatic stress disorder (PTSD) and the other anxiety disorders is that:
   a. the person experiences acute anxiety with feelings of panic.
   b. the person has physiological reactions, not just psychological ones.
   c. Prozac usually works best with PTSD.
   d. symptoms begin after exposure to a traumatic stressor.

3. All except which of the following occur during the sympathetic response (or the fight-or-flight reaction) to a stressor?
   a. Heart rate and blood pressure increase.
   b. Breathing rate increases.
   c. Blood clotting ability decreases.
   d. Immune responses decrease.

4. Sharon is admitted for an appendectomy. As you enter the room to prep Sharon for surgery, she is breathing rapidly, sweating, restless, and anxious. Your most therapeutic intervention at this time would be to:
   a. provide Sharon with information about her surgery, telling her what to expect when she comes out of the recovery room.

NURSING PROCESS WORKSHEET

Health Problem (Title)

Client Goal*

Related to

↓

Etiology (Related Factors)

Nursing Interventions**

Evidenced by

↓

**Signs and Symptoms
(Defining Characteristics)**

Evaluative Statement

*More than one client goal may be appropriate. For this exercise, choose one client goal that demonstrates a direct resolution of the client problem identified in the nursing diagnosis.

**Be sure you are able to list the scientific rationale for each nursing intervention you order.

b. speak to Sharon with simple, short directions in a soothing voice, and do not ask her to make choices about positioning or comfort.

c. provide Sharon with instructions; however, provide very limited choices about positioning/comfort measures.

d. leave the room, providing silence for Sharon until she regains her composure.

5. All except which of the following brain structures are known to play a role in the anxiety disorders?

a. Amygdala

b. Hippocampus

c. Locus ceruleus

d. Cerebellum

6. One of the major differences between generalized anxiety disorder (GAD) and panic disorder is that:

a. in GAD, the person usually does not experience eruptions of acute anxiety.

b. in panic disorder, the person suffers from a chronic state of elevated anxiety.

c. panic disorders are more easily treated than GAD.

d. GAD is characterized by occasional, unexpected panic attacks.

7. Which of the following is often a comorbid condition with anxiety disorders?

a. High alcohol intake or use of illicit mood-altering drugs

b. A history of severe trauma in childhood

c. A mother who was overly involved and had difficulty with boundaries

d. A history of depression

8. The nurse asks Jonathan, a 25-year-old man with panic attacks, to role-play a situation in which Jonathan is in the grocery store and is beginning to have an attack. This is considered what type of intervention?

a. Cognitive therapy, using covert rehearsal

b. Cognitive behavioral therapy, using cognitive reframing

c. Systematic desensitization treatment

d. Relaxation retraining

9. When Jonathan is placed on fluoxetine (Prozac), the therapist is certain to explain that:

a. sometimes in the first week of treatment, you may experience heightened feelings of anxiety, but these will pass when you become accustomed to the new medication.

b. this medication can cause addiction, so you need to keep the doses constant.

c. you may experience dry mouth and drowsiness during the first 2 days of treatment.

d. this medication takes up to 3 months to be effective, so be patient.

10. Jonathan comes in for a therapy session and is having a mild panic attack. The therapist asks him to relax in his chair and then gently asks him to imagine himself in a very safe and calm place. This technique, often useful in anxiety disorders, is called:

a. cognitive therapy.

b. desensitization.

c. visualization.

d. problem-solving.

CHAPTER 19

The Client With a Somatoform Disorder

Somatoform disorders are characterized by client complaints of severe physical symptoms or disability that are not explained readily by organic or physical pathology on testing or examination. Somatoform disorders must be distinguished from psychological factors affecting medical conditions, in which an identifiable medical illness is associated with psychological factors (eg, depression, anxiety). Somatoform disorders are approximately 10 times more common in women than in men, with the first symptoms usually appearing in adolescence.

This group of disorders result from unconscious processes in which clients use physical symptoms to express emotional needs, such as gaining attention and forcing others to meet their dependency needs.

Clients with somatoform disorders have highly elaborate self-diagnoses and symptoms that are not responsive to reassurance, explanation, or standard treatment. Symptoms associated with somatoform disorders often unconsciously enable the client to assume the "sick role," which relieves him or her of social obligations and responsibilities and meets his or her dependency needs.

Somatoform disorders are very difficult to treat and require an interdisciplinary, chronic care approach. Clinical treatments consist of individual, group, and family psychotherapy and a selection of limited somatic therapies, most often SSRIs.

Using the nursing process with a client with a somatoform disorder involves assessing the client on a psychological, physiological, and social level, determining nursing diagnoses, planning care, implementing care, and evaluating the treatment plan. Frequent and ongoing evaluation of the treatment plan and the client's response to interventions is critical to assist the client to move toward the goals of increased health and well-being and optimal functional status.

LEARNING OBJECTIVES

After completing the exercises in this workbook, and studying the corresponding chapter in the textbook, the student will be able to:

- Define the term "somatoform disorder."

- Differentiate somatoform disorders from organic physical disorders influenced by psychological factors.

- Discuss the epidemiology of somatoform disorders, including prevalence, gender, and age of onset.

- Describe possible psychological, neurobiological, and familial etiologies of somatoform disorders.

- Describe signs and symptoms of somatoform disorders.

- Identify the most common interdisciplinary goals and treatments for clients with somatoform disorders.

- Apply the steps of the nursing process—assessment, nursing diagnosis, planning, implementation, and evaluation—to clients who exhibit somatoform disorders.

KEY TERMS

Body dysmorphic disorder: A somatoform disorder in which the client is preoccupied with an imagined defect in his or her appearance (eg, a facial flaw or spot) when no abnormality or disturbance actually exists.

Conversion disorder: A somatoform disorder in which the client has at least one symptom or deficit of sensory or voluntary motor function (eg, paralysis) that cannot be explained by a neurological or general medical condition.

Culture-bound syndromes: Forms of mental illness found in only one particular culture, symbolizing that culture's unique expression of physical or mental distress.

Hypervigilance: A common symptom of somatoform disorders in which the client's heightened focus on the body and its sensations leads to chronic, prolonged misinterpretation and overreaction to physical signs.

Hypochondriasis: A somatoform disorder characterized by a client's unwarranted fear or belief that he or she has a serious disease, without significant pathology.

Hysteria: An historical term (preceding somatoform disorder) coined in the early 1900s by Sigmund Freud to describe a condition in which people could not use certain body parts despite having no physiological damage or dysfunction.

La belle indifference: In conversion disorder, a remarkable lack of affect or concern shown by a client despite a symptom that imposes significant physical disability (eg, paralysis).

Primary gain: The main benefit a person derives from the "sick role," which, in the case of somatoform disorders, is the blocking of psychological conflict from conscious awareness.

Psychosomatic medicine: The clinical and scientific study of the connections between the mind and body.

Secondary gain: Additional benefits that a person derives from the "sick role"; examples include being released from expected responsibilities and receiving attention from others.

Sick role: The role that all chronically ill clients assume that releases them from usual responsibilities; in somatoform disorders, clients unconsciously assume the sick role to meet their dependency needs.

Somatization disorder: A somatoform disorder characterized by many physical complaints over several years that cannot be explained by pathology or a general medical condition.

Somatoform disorders: A group of psychiatric disorders in which clients complain of extreme physiologic discomfort or disability without any identifiable pathology on testing or examination.

Chapter Outline

SOMATOFORM DISORDERS
Epidemiology
Cultural Considerations
Etiology
Signs and Symptoms/Diagnostic Criteria
Primary and Secondary Gain
Somatization Disorder
Undifferentiated Somatoform Disorder
Conversion Disorder
Pain Disorder
Hypochondriasis
Body Dysmorphic Disorder
Somatoform Disorder Not Otherwise Specified (NOS)
Comorbidities and Dual Diagnoses
Implications and Prognosis
Interdisciplinary Goals and Treatment

Individual and Group Psychotherapies
Somatic Therapies
APPLICATION OF THE NURSING PROCESS TO THE CLIENT WITH A SOMATOFORM DISORDER
Assessment
Psychological Assessment
  Behavior
  Mood and Affect
  Thought Process and Content
  Intellectual and Cognitive Processing
  Insight and Judgment
  Suicidal Ideation
Physical Examination
  Vegetative Signs
  Energy and Psychomotor Functioning
Social Assessment
Nursing Diagnoses
Planning
Implementation
Establishing a Trusting Relationship
Managing Ineffective Coping
Addressing Powerlessness and Dependency Issues
Enhancing Self-Esteem
Reducing Anxiety
Re-establishing Social Activities
Re-establishing Functional Family Processes
Evaluation

KEY TOPICS

Somatoform Disorders: Epidemiology, etiology, signs and symptoms, comorbidities, dual diagnoses, implications and prognosis, interdisciplinary treatments.

Nursing Process: Assessment (psychological, physiological, social); diagnosis, planning, implementation (establishing trust, managing coping, enhancing self-esteem, reducing anxiety), evaluation

■ Exercises

CASE STUDY EXERCISE

Cindy S., age 45, lives with her husband of 25 years. She has four grown children, three boys and one girl. Cindy comes to the psychiatric advanced practice registered nurse on a referral from her physician, who says, "I have tried everything I know how to do, but I just can't seem to help Cindy feel better. She has no demonstrable physiologic problems, and I've given her several "million-dollar" workups in the last 2 years. I'm beginning to think it's something psychological." On Cindy's first visit, she monopolizes the session with a litany of physical complaints, including five abdominal surgeries for pain of unknown origin, three recent intravenous pyelograms due to kidney pain with no known etiology, and a long history of visiting numerous physicians in many specialty areas. She states, "This all started when I was 20 and I got a gastrointestinal blockage. Since then, I've had numbness in my stomach area, and I've really had trouble with light in my eyes, because it makes me unsteady and I feel like I'm going to fall down." She states, "I'm at my wit's end! I can't stand this anymore. None of these doctors know what they're doing, and I'm still hurting really bad. I can't even get out of my house! And don't try and tell me it's all in my head, either. Because I know I have pain, and I have a feeling that I will eventually die of cancer."

1. In this first visit, the goal of the nurse therapist is to establish a therapeutic relationship with Cindy. Using the direct quotations from Cindy during this interview, discuss some therapeutic communication responses that will assist the therapist to achieve this goal.

On subsequent visits with the therapist, Cindy reveals that her husband, Randy, has been a supportive and loving husband. She expresses guilt over her illness and that she has "made Randy stay home every day and take care of me instead of going out with friends." She is also very sad about her four children, none of whom have met her expectations for their lives thus far. She expresses that she has been a "terrible mother, and I obviously have no clue about how to raise decent children." In fact, Cindy's children are all high-functioning, responsible professionals with families.

2. Barsky & Borus (1999) spoke of four psychosocial factors that seem to propel the cycle of symptom exaggeration in somatoform disorders (of which somatization disorder is one). Discuss these factors, and provide evidence of Cindy's experience of each one.

3. List symptoms that provide evidence that Cindy is suffering from somatization disorder.

4. List some assessment questions that you would plan to ask Cindy's husband, Randy.

After 6 months of weekly therapy sessions, Cindy is beginning to somatize less and to focus more on outside activities, and she has begun to go to the YMCA swimming pool once a week. The therapist is using a variety of treatment approaches that have been helping Cindy to refocus her attention toward her feelings and away from her body.

5. Discuss overarching interventions that are useful for treating clients such as Cindy. Explain why each of these interventions helps with somatizing clients.

6. Describe specific therapeutic interventions that might help Cindy to focus her attention away from her physical complaints and more toward her psychological and emotional issues.

7. Taking all of the data given in the above case study scenario, complete the Nursing Process Worksheet on the next page, planning care for Cindy that includes specific individual goals as well as goals for overarching care management.

CRITICAL THINKING AND SELF-EVALUATION EXERCISES

1. Have you ever had the experience of listening to another person talk about his or her physical condition excessively? What was the circumstance? How might this experience be different from working with a client who has a somatoform disorder?

2. If you were in extreme pain, describe some of the things a loved one could do or say that might ease your pain. Explain how these things would help to alleviate your pain.

■ NCLEX-Style Exam Questions

1. In somatoform disorders, all except which of the following are true?
   a. The client believes he/she has a serious illness.
   b. The client embraces the "sick role."
   c. The client believes that his/her condition is catastrophic and disabling.
   d. The client usually believes he/she has some sort of anxiety disorder.

NURSING PROCESS WORKSHEET

Health Problem (Title)

Client Goal*

Related to

↓

Etiology (Related Factors)

Nursing Interventions**

Evidenced by

↓

**Signs and Symptoms
(Defining Characteristics)**

Evaluative Statement

*More than one client goal may be appropriate. For this exercise, choose one client goal that demonstrates a direct resolution of the client problem identified in the nursing diagnosis.

**Be sure you are able to list the scientific rationale for each nursing intervention you order.

2. *Hwa-byung* is a Korean syndrome that:

   a. is characterized by suppressed anger, leading to indigestion, anorexia, fatigue, and other aches and pains.

   b. is characterized by symptoms of loss of concentration, dizziness, and headaches.

   c. occurs primarily in adolescents and leads to decreased memory, concentration, and cognitive ability.

   d. involves a generalized stress response that includes crying, fainting, and a total loss of control.

3. What is the major clinical finding in somatoform disorders?

   a. The report of symptoms with no demonstrable pathology on testing or examination

   b. The client's inability to focus on emotional content

   c. Pain with a history of "doctor-shopping"

   d. Loss of voluntary motor or sensory functioning

4. Which of the following is a significant obstacle in providing psychiatric care for clients who have somatoform disorders?

   a. They are often unrecognized because clients receive treatment in different primary care offices, and care is often fragmented.

   b. Clients with these disorders find it difficult to go to a clinic setting.

   c. Clients are often embarrassed about the number and extent of their physical complaints.

   d. There are no known successful treatments for these disorders.

5. Medications have been tried for somatization disorder. Which of the following drugs have been shown to be effective in some cases?

   a. Antipsychotics

   b. SSRIs

   c. Antianxiety agents

   d. Antihypertensive drugs

6. The therapist working with a client who is suffering from a somatization disorder may use a variety of therapeutic techniques. Which of the following is an intervention that could be carried out by a generalist registered nurse?

   a. Conduct psychotherapy that focuses on helping the client to express needs in terms of verbal requests and not focusing on bodily symptoms

   b. Consult with the client's physicians, discuss the client's broad treatment plan, and plan for an interdisciplinary approach to outpatient treatment over time

   c. Conduct a training session with primary care physicians regarding how to manage the somatizing client in private practice

   d. Develop trust, establish a therapeutic relationship, and assist the client with stress-management techniques

7. Steven has somatization disorder and is complaining of back pain that will not stop. You are in the working phase of the therapeutic relationship. He has recently been fired from his job of 10 years due to missing work. What is the most therapeutic nursing intervention with Steven at this point?

   a. "Steven, I really think that your back pain is just an excuse to avoid the fact that you were fired."

   b. "Steven, how is it that you got fired? I didn't realize you were missing that much work."

   c. "Steven, I understand that your back is hurting. Do you feel there may be some sort of connection between your recent difficulties at work and your increased back pain?"

   d. "Back pain is very uncomfortable. Perhaps we should seek an x-ray with your medical doctor to rule out any physical problems."

8. You are admitting Cheryl, who has panic disorder, to the inpatient unit. On your admission interview, Cheryl appears to be in the middle of one of the panic attacks that frequently occur—she is diaphoretic, wringing her hands, gasping, and darting her eyes around the room, and she appears flushed. She states she doesn't know what's wrong and can't seem to calm down. What is the most therapeutic nursing intervention at this time?

   a. "Cheryl, please try and concentrate, as I need to ask a couple of very important questions." Then ask only the essential elements of the admission interview.

   b. "Cheryl, I can see you are anxious. Why don't I take you on a unit tour instead of being cooped up in this room."

   c. "Cheryl, it seems that you may be having a panic attack. Let's stop the interview for now. Just sit back and relax in the chair, and take a few deep breaths."

   d. "Cheryl, can I offer you some Valium? I think it may help you right now."

9. In the above question, which of the following would be an appropriate nursing diagnosis?
   a. Anxiety related to feelings about admission and/or intake interview, as evidenced by diaphoresis, flushing, wringing of hands, and gasping
   b. Ineffective Coping related to inability to trust, evidenced by eyes darting around room
   c. Social Isolation related to being alone in interview room, evidenced by panic attack during interview
   d. Powerlessness related to being interviewed, evidenced by attempting to gain control through use of a panic attack

10. Which of the following questions would NOT be helpful in eliciting information about family influences in somatoform disorders?
   a. Have any of the client's family members used similar behavior to the client's when adapting to stress?
   b. Did the client grow up in a family that expressed physical illnesses or symptoms frequently?
   c. What roles have changed in the family because of the client's illness?
   d. Have any of the client's family members ever been arrested for domestic disturbance?

CHAPTER 20

The Client With a Sexual or Gender Disorder

To work professionally and to avoid applying his or her own biases to clients, the nurse must be aware of his or her own views and learn about the views of the client populations with whom he or she works. Kaplan has identified three phases of the human sexual response: desire, excitement, and orgasm. Sexual dysfunction disorders can be primary or secondary. General medical conditions and substance use may affect sexual interest and abilities.

Treatment of specific sexual dysfunctions focuses mainly on targeting the client and contributing causal factors related to the particular disorder. Generalist nurses provide education and counseling for clients seeking help with sexual dysfunction. Nurses encourage clients seeking help for sexual dysfunction to express their feelings surrounding the problem. They should assess and address self-esteem issues.

"Paraphilias" refer to those sexual expressions characterized by recurrent, intense sexually arousing fantasies, urges, or behaviors. They persist over at least 6 months. Several types of paraphilias include exhibitionism, fetishism, frotteurism, pedophilia, sexual masochism, sexual sadism, transvestic fetishism, and voyeurism.

Gender identity manifests differently in children and adolescents/adults. Children may repeatedly state a desire to be, or insist that they are, the other sex. In adolescents and adults, the disturbance is manifested by symptoms such as a stated desire to be the other sex, frequent "passing" as the other sex, desire to live or be treated as the other sex, or the conviction that they have the typical feelings and reactions of the other sex.

LEARNING OBJECTIVES

After completing the exercises in this workbook, and studying the corresponding chapter in the textbook, the student will be able to:

- Recognize his or her own sexual beliefs and values to avoid imposing them on clients.

- Describe the factors that affect sexual expression.

- Discuss the phases of human sexual response.

- Understand the various methods of achieving orgasm.

- Describe normal age-related sexual changes.

- Discuss the causes of sexual dysfunction disorders.

- Describe the treatment approaches for sexual dysfunction disorders.

- Apply the nursing process to the care of a client with a sexual dysfunction.

- Discuss the types of paraphilias.

- Compare and contrast the signs and symptoms of gender identity disorders as they manifest in children and adults.

KEY TERMS

Arousal: Physiological stimulation, such as touching, kissing, fondling, licking, or biting erogenous body parts, that causes changes in the genitals.

Bisexuality: An equal or almost equal attraction to or preference for either sex as a sexual partner.

Desire: Activation of areas in the brain that produce sexual appetite or drive.

Dyspareunia: Genital pain associated with sexual intercourse in either a man or woman.

Excitement: Psychological stimulation during the desire phase such as sexual fantasies or romantic communication.

Foreplay: Petting and fondling behaviors that cause arousal during the excitement phase.

Heterosexuality: An attraction to and preference for members of the opposite sex as sexual partners.

Homosexuality: An attraction to and preference for members of the same sex as sexual partners.

Masturbation: Self-stimulation of erogenous areas to the point of orgasm.

Orgasm: The peak of sexual pleasure. In the female it consists of 3 to 15 strong rhythmic contractions of the orgasmic platform of the vagina. In the male, it consists of emission and ejaculation.

Paraphilias: Sexual expressions for at least 6 months that are characterized by recurrent, intense sexual urges, fantasies, or behaviors that generally involve nonhuman objects or animals, suffering or humiliation of self or partner, or children or other nonconsenting persons.

Premature ejaculation: A persistent or recurrent onset of orgasm and ejaculation with minimal sexual stimulation before, on, or shortly after penetration and before the person wishes it.

Sexual dysfunction: Sexual expressions characterized by a disturbance in the processes that characterize the sexual response cycle or by pain associated with sexual intercourse.

Sexual intercourse (coitus): Penetration of the vagina by the penis.

Sexuality: The experience of the sexual self.

Transsexual: A person who identifies with and lives as if he or she is of the opposite gender.

Transvestite: A person who cross-dresses for the purpose of sexual arousal.

Vaginismus: Recurrent or persistent involuntary spasm of the musculature of the outer third of the vagina, which interferes with sexual intercourse.

Chapter Outline

NORMAL HUMAN SEXUALITY
Sexual Expression
Effects of Sexual Orientation on Sexual Expression
Sexual Preference
Gender Role
Sexual Identity
Effects of Culture on Sexual Expression
Effects of Ill Health on Sexual Expression
Sexual Response
Human Sexual Response Phases
Desire
Excitement
Orgasm
Normal Age-Related Sexual Changes
SEXUAL AND GENDER DISORDERS
SEXUAL DYSFUNCTION DISORDERS
Etiology
Signs and Symptoms/Diagnostic Criteria
Desire Disorders
Arousal Disorders
Orgasmic Disorders
Pain Disorders

Interdisciplinary Goals and Treatments
Pharmacological Therapy
Sex Therapy
APPLICATION OF THE NURSING PROCESS TO THE CLIENT WITH SEXUAL DYSFUNCTION
Assessment
Nursing Diagnosis
Planning
Implementation
Counseling the Client with a Sexual Dysfunction Disorder
Enhancing Self-Esteem
Evaluation
PARAPHILIAS
Signs and Symptoms/Diagnostic Criteria
Interdisciplinary Goals and Treatment
GENDER IDENTITY DISORDERS
Signs and Symptoms/Diagnostic Criteria
Interdisciplinary Goals and Treatment
Sex Reassignment Surgery
Hormone Treatment
Psychotherapy

KEY TOPICS

Normal human sexuality: Sexual expression (sexual orientation, preference, gender role, sexual identity); sexual response (desire, excitement, orgasm)

Sexual and gender disorders: Sexual dysfunction disorders (disorders of desire, arousal, orgasm, pain)

Nursing process: Assessment, diagnosis, planning, implementation (counseling, enhancing self-esteem)

Paraphilias, Gender Identity Disorders

■ Exercises

CASE STUDY EXERCISE

This case study is designed to illustrate issues that are commonly seen in individuals who are exploring and coming to terms with their sexuality, particularly homosexuality. Remember that homosexuality is a sexual preference, not a psychiatric diagnosis. However, it is not uncommon to see young men and women admitted to psychiatric inpatient units for depression, anxiety, or suicidal behavior that may be precipitated or exacerbated by the struggle to recognize and embrace their sexual preference in a society in which that preference is stigmatized and rejected. Young men and women very often find themselves isolated, alone, and virtually cut off from long-standing family and friends because of their emerging preference for same-sex partners. Some individuals make an attempt to reject their homosexuality and embrace a heterosexual lifestyle, which can create internal dissonance and depression in the person over time. It is important for nurses in all areas of healthcare to recognize and to be able to respond therapeutically to individuals who are homosexual. In addition, nurses must be aware of their own feelings and biases around sexuality in general, and around specific sexual issues such as homosexuality, in order to recognize when personal values may affect the treatment of a client.

Jim T., age 26, has been admitted to the psychiatric inpatient unit for depression following an argument yesterday with his parents in which he told them he was homosexual. Following the argument, Jim was found by his partner, Ted, in the bedroom of their apartment attempting to take an overdose of Tylenol. Jim had taken 10 Tylenol tablets when Ted found him, and Ted immediately took him to the emergency room. Jim was found to be suicidal in the ER and was transferred for a brief inpatient stay in psychiatry.

Jim is employed full-time as a computer technologist at a local bank and does well in his position. Jim was raised in a Baptist family where church attendance each week was a staple of family life. Both parents are very active in the community as well. Jim dated several girls in high school because he felt he needed to try to "do the right thing," but he realized that he was very uncomfortable having sexual relations with women and would often have anxiety episodes during those relationships. When he entered college, he began to explore his sexuality more freely and realized that he was homosexual. He has struggled with issues of low self-esteem since then, often feeling that he is "no good to anybody."

He had not "come out" to his family before now because he had not had anyone in his life who was significant. However, for the past year, he has been dating Ted, and the two men have committed to be life partners. Jim spoke with his parents in the hope that they might be accepting and might embrace Ted into the family as well. When Jim told his parents, they both were shocked and expressed their outrage and disappointment with him as a person, and with his lifestyle. They asked him never to bring Ted to their home and told him that if he persisted with this

"sin against God," he would no longer be welcomed either.

Jim cries as he tells you, his admitting nurse, about the argument. He is very sad about the events and has been contemplating suicide. However, he states, "I just can't do that, because it would hurt Ted too much." (For the purposes of this chapter, the following questions will focus on issues of sexuality, instead of assessing for depression and suicidal ideation, topics covered in other chapters.)

1. In an attempt to learn more about Jim's sexuality, and using Textbook Table 20-3, list what types of questions might elicit the information that you would need to make a comprehensive sexuality assessment.

After 2 days on the unit, Jim appears brighter and is very talkative and active in the milieu. He has not received medications since his admission and states, "I think I can get through this without medication. I've never been depressed before, and this is really specific to my recent issues with myself and the family." He is no longer suicidal and has begun to focus on issues around his current relationship with Ted. He continues to express sadness regarding his family; however, he is interested in exploring how he can help himself to be more comfortable with his life and his homosexuality.

2. To work with Jim regarding his issues around homosexuality, you first need to assess his history. Provide examples of questions you could ask to assess his homosexual history.

3. Are there ways in which you might work with Jim and his boyfriend while Jim is admitted? What might you discuss with them?

4. What are your thoughts about medications for Jim? Explain your opinions about whether or not you think Jim should take medications, and provide rationales for your opinions.

5. Develop a Nursing Process Worksheet for Jim's care at this point, using data you have gathered so far in the case study. Develop at least two nursing diagnoses.

NURSING PROCESS WORKSHEET

Health Problem (Title)

Client Goal*

Related to

↓

Etiology (Related Factors)

Nursing Interventions**

Evidenced by

↓

**Signs and Symptoms
(Defining Characteristics)**

Evaluative Statement

*More than one client goal may be appropriate. For this exercise, choose one client goal that demonstrates a direct resolution of the client problem identified in the nursing diagnosis.

**Be sure you are able to list the scientific rationale for each nursing intervention you order.

As Jim prepares for discharge, he says, "You know, Ted and I have never been tested for HIV. I'm a little worried, because I had multiple partners before meeting Ted, and I know he did too."

6. Discuss how you would respond to this statement.

7. What could you teach Jim about safer sex options for physical intimacy?

CRITICAL THINKING AND SELF-EVALUATION EXERCISES

1. Reflect on how you would feel if you were assigned to care for Jim in the above scenario. Be as honest with yourself as possible. Explore your feelings about sexual preference, and identify any biases or issues that you feel might impede your work with clients who are experiencing sexual difficulties of any type. Discuss how these feelings might bias your work and how you might overcome it.

2. Which of the sexual disorders do you believe would be most difficult for you to work with? Think and reflect on reasons why it would be more difficult. Develop strategies you might use if you encounter clients with this disorder in your practice.

■ NCLEX-Style Exam Questions

1. Laura comes to her primary care physician complaining of extreme pain upon intercourse. She states that this is causing discomfort and anger between her and her husband of 6 months. Laura is suffering from
   a. dissociative identity disorder.
   b. dyspareunia.
   c. paraphilia.
   d. vaginismus.

2. Research has shown, in regard to homosexuals and bisexuals, that
   a. their sexual behavior varies as much as that of heterosexuals.
   b. pedophilia and promiscuity are more prevalent than in heterosexuals.
   c. they tend to stay with one partner longer than do heterosexuals.
   d. their marriages are now legally recognized in 46 states.

3. Which of the following is an example of "sexual acting-out behaviors" exhibited by a male client toward a female nurse?
   a. The male client asks the female nurse to help with his bed bath.
   b. The male client seeks the female nurse out when he needs to use the restroom.
   c. The male client asks the female nurse to check on a rash he has developed on his scrotum.
   d. The male client pats the female nurse on the buttock as she turns to leave the room.

4. Susan, an RN, is taking care of John, age 22, who is 3 days postop from an emergency appendectomy. As she enters John's room at 11 pm, she abruptly stops as she sees that John is masturbating. The following is the most therapeutic nursing intervention:
   a. "John, that will cause your incision to open and is not really appropriate here."
   b. "John, your behavior is inappropriate and may be disturbing to other clients."
   c. "Oh, my! I can't believe you're doing that here!"
   d. "Excuse me, John. Let me pull your curtain, and I'll be back later to check on you."

5. The sexual dysfunction disorders are broken into the following subgroups:
   a. desire, arousal, orgasmic, and pain disorders.
   b. desire, arousal, orgasmic, and gender conflict disorders.
   c. lifelong, acquired, generalized, or situational disorders.
   d. primary, secondary, arousal, and orgasmic disorders.

6. Roman, age 36, is single. He comes to the physician complaining of inability to attain or maintain an erection. Which of the following would be the most therapeutic nursing intervention?
   a. "Roman, you have hypoactive sexual disorder, and there are several medications that may be helpful."
   b. "Roman, don't worry about this. There are many men who go through phases of not being able to maintain an erection, and these are usually short-lived."
   c. "Roman, you may have sexual aversion disorder. Have you noticed that you have anxi-

ety when you are with your partner in an intimate situation?"

d. "Roman, it sounds like you may have erectile dysfunction. It may be helpful to try a course of sildenafil citrate (Viagra) to see if it would help you."

7. When assessing an individual for sexual dysfunction, it is most therapeutic for the nurse to

a. frame questions in a way that normalizes a wide range of sexual behaviors and problems and use terms that the client will understand.

b. use his/her own experience as a background for selecting specific questions, and to ask questions with which the nurse is most familiar and comfortable.

c. assume that most clients are fairly comfortable discussing their sexuality, especially if they are married.

d. avoid addressing various lifestyle concerns, particularly with gay clients, because this can cause a great deal of discomfort and even shutdown during the interview.

8. One of the most common nursing diagnoses for clients who are experiencing sexual dysfunction is

a. ineffective family coping related to difficulty with sexual pleasure.

b. ineffective sexuality pattern related to desire, arousal, orgasmic, or pain disorder.

c. potential for depressive illness related to sadness about lack of sexual ability.

d. situational low self-esteem related to withdrawal of partner from intimacy.

9. Thomas, age 40, has been diagnosed with a paraphilia. All except which of the following are paraphilias?

a. Exhibitionism

b. Fetishism

c. Frotteurism

d. Dyspareunia

10. Thomas has complained of recurrent impulses to go to the local mall and touch or rub up against people who are shopping or standing in line. He states that although this is fairly easy to do, he becomes embarrassed as he becomes erect during this activity and occasionally has an ejaculation, which is "very humiliating." From the clinical information above, which of the paraphilias is Thomas suffering from?

a. Exhibitionism

b. Dyspareunia

c. Fetishism

d. Frotteurism

CHAPTER 21

The Client With a Dissociative Disorder

Dissociative disorders are thought by some scholars to be caused by trauma; the individual attempts to deal with this trauma by escaping into the mind. Behaviors of the person, however, are dysfunctional. Types of dissociative disorders include depersonalization disorder, dissociative amnesia, dissociative fugue, and dissociative identity disorder (DID, formerly called multiple personality disorder). The most severe of the dissociative disorders is DID.

Treatment modalities for dissociative disorders may include individual and group therapy, art therapy, and milieu management. The nursing assessment for DID should include detailed questions about the client's family history and the client's present level of functioning. The nurse must consider the total client picture because many clients with DID have been misdiagnosed, as symptoms were treated independently. Nursing diagnoses include attention to the client's safety, level of anxiety, coping mechanisms, self-esteem, role performance, and multiple personality fragments. Planning the client's treatment involves collaboration with the client and other disciplines. Goals include assisting the client with learning new coping strategies and, in DID, reintegrating the client's personality as much as possible.

Interventions for clients with DID include providing a consistent milieu for client safety, holding the client responsible for the behaviors of all alters, teaching the client "grounding" techniques, and providing the client with opportunities to practice new coping strategies prior to discharge. Recovery may be evaluated by the client's functional level.

LEARNING OBJECTIVES

After completing the exercises in this workbook, and studying the corresponding chapter in the textbook, the student will be able to:

- Define "dissociation."

- Describe the etiology of dissociative disorders.

- Differentiate the four types of dissociative disorders.

- Describe addictions commonly associated with dissociative disorders.

- Describe treatment modalities for dissociative disorders.

- Apply the nursing process to clients with dissociative disorders.

- Understand cultural considerations applicable to the care of clients with dissociative disorders.

KEY TERMS

Alter: Two or more identities or personality states.

Depersonalization disorder: A dissociative disorder characterized by a recurring or persistent feeling that one is detached from one's own thinking. Affected clients feel that they are outside their mind or body, much like an observer.

Dissociation: Altering one's usual level of self-awareness in an effort to escape an upsetting event or feeling.

Dissociative amnesia: A dissociative disorder characterized by loss of memory that is not organic and involves an inability to recall events or facts too extensive to be labeled as mere forgetfulness.

Dissociative disorder: A disruption in the usually integrated functions of consciousness, memory, identity, or perception, causing a disturbance that may be sudden or gradual, transient or chronic.

Dissociative fugue: A dissociative disorder that involves sudden travel away from home coupled with an inability to remember the past and confusion about identity or the adoption of a new identity.

Dissociative identity disorder: A dissociative disorder in which the person acquires two or more identities or personality states (alters), who take control over the client's behavior.

Dissociative trance: A dissociative state in which a person's awareness of his or her immediate surroundings narrows, and he or she exhibits stereotyped behaviors such as immobilization, collapse, or uncontrollable shrieking.

Possession trance: A dissociative state that involves acquiring a new identity attributed to the influence of a spirit, power, deity, or other person.

Ritual abuse: A severe form of abuse in which a child is repeatedly physically and sexually abused in ceremonies by an organized group of perpetrators.

Chapter Outline

DISSOCIATIVE DISORDERS
Epidemiology
Cultural Considerations
Etiology
Biologic Factors
Psychological and Social Factors
Role of Family Dynamics
Signs and Symptoms/Diagnostic Criteria
Comorbidities and Dual Diagnoses
Interdisciplinary Goals and Treatment
Treatment Approach
Individual Therapy for Dissociative Disorders
Group Therapy
Pharmacotherapy
Art Therapy
Milieu Management
Family Education
APPLICATION OF THE NURSING PROCESS TO THE CLIENT WITH A DISSOCIATIVE DISORDER
Assessment in Adults
Assessment in Children
Nursing Diagnosis
Planning
Implementation
Evaluation

KEY TOPICS

Dissociative disorder: Biologic, psychological, and social factors; role of family dynamics

Interdisciplinary goals and treatments: Individual, group, art therapies; pharmacotherapy; milieu management; family education

Nursing process: Assessment of adults; assessment of children; diagnosis; planning; implementation; evaluation

■ Exercises

CASE STUDY EXERCISE

Laurie, age 22, was admitted last night to the inpatient psychiatric unit after she was found by her mother sobbing in her bedroom at home and saying, "I just can't take this anymore. I'm really, really sad, Mom." She has just completed her B.S.

degree and is living at home for the summer. When the nurse interviews Laurie, she states, "I always feel sort of separate from the room I'm in. I mean, it's really hard to describe, but I feel like I'm outside looking in. I feel like I'm watching myself think and talk. Oh, I know how to describe it to you—have you ever been driving and you get mesmerized and then don't even remember going through a certain section of town on the way home? Well, that's how I feel almost every day. It started when I was 18 with one or two times a month, but these feelings have gradually taken over most of my day. It was hard to get through college, and I don't know how I did it. But now, since I've come home to Mom and Dad's house, it is really starting to get in my way. I need to go out looking for a job, but I just don't feel like I can concentrate. I feel so sad and depressed about it, like it will never end."

1. On a continuum of dissociation (see Textbook, Fig. 21-1), where do you think Laurie falls? Explain why.

2. How would you describe, in professional terms, Laurie's description of driving and become mesmerized?

On the initial admission assessment, Laurie also reveals that she has had thoughts of cutting her arm "to bring me back to reality." Although she has never done so, she believes this may help her to refocus when she is dissociating.

3. Discuss the areas of assessment you will cover during Laurie's admission interview. Provide examples of therapeutic nursing questions that will help you to assess Laurie's behaviors, thoughts, and perceptions. Frame your questions specifically for Laurie (do not use standardized, generic questions).

4. Develop a Nursing Process Worksheet to address the most important nursing concern during Laurie's first 24 hours on your unit.

During Laurie's first week on the unit, she says, "Since I've been here, I think I have been able to stay with people while I'm talking. It feels good. It's more like I was about a year ago." She is participating in the milieu, although she tends to remain on

NURSING PROCESS WORKSHEET

Health Problem (Title)

Client Goal*

Related to

↓

Etiology (Related Factors)

Nursing Interventions**

Evidenced by

↓

**Signs and Symptoms
(Defining Characteristics)**

Evaluative Statement

*More than one client goal may be appropriate. For this exercise, choose one client goal that demonstrates a direct resolution of the client problem identified in the nursing diagnosis.
**Be sure you are able to list the scientific rationale for each nursing intervention you order.

the edge of groups and rather silent in groups. However, you are noticing a difference in her energy level and in her discussions with you. She appears to remain on target with her discussions and stays engaged in the conversation much more closely than she did upon admission.

5. As Laurie's primary nurse, you are developing ideas about ways you can support the gains Laurie has made over the past week. Describe some techniques you can use to accomplish this goal.

Laurie has been on the unit for 3 weeks and reports feeling significantly better. Her behavior has evolved from total withdrawal to participating more actively with friends she has made on the unit and in groups and activities. The plan is to discharge Laurie to home the following day.

6. List and discuss three major goals for Laurie's discharge planning.

CRITICAL THINKING AND SELF-EVALUATION EXERCISES

1. Imagine that you are Laurie's primary nurse. Discuss some of the ideas you have about her behaviors and thoughts. Do these invoke any feelings within yourself?

2. To what extent, if any, do you have an understanding of Laurie's symptoms and disorder? Would you be able to empathize with her, and to provide therapeutic care? Why or why not?

▪ NCLEX-Style Exam Questions

1. Historically, dissociative disorders
   a. were discovered in the early 1960s and have never been considered legitimate phenomena by the scientific community.
   b. were considered deviant behavior that required the individual to be placed in jail in the mid-1950s.
   c. have come under closer scrutiny in recent years and are gaining acceptance as clinically legitimate phenomena.
   d. were placed in the category of depressive disorders and thus were not recognized in clinical practice until recently.

2. Joan describes an 8-hour drive to visit her relatives in another state and says that she does not remember much of the road trip and can't believe she arrived safely. This phenomenon is best described as
   a. dissociative amnesia.
   b. dissociative fugue.
   c. dissociative identity disorder.
   d. dissociative state.

3. People with dissociative disorders:
   a. are, for the most part, not easily hypnotizable.
   b. usually have an underlying depression that is causing them to dissociate.
   c. are unusual in their ability to lie to others without ethical worries.
   d. are particularly sensitive to hypnotism, are highly suggestible, and have low sedation thresholds.

4. All except which of the following are considered "dissociative disorders"?
   a. Dissociative state
   b. Dissociative fugue
   c. Depersonalization disorder
   d. Dissociative amnesia

5. The major, overarching nursing goal for treatment of the client with dissociative identity disorder (DID) is
   a. absence of all dissociative episodes from the client's conscious awareness.
   b. integration of all of the client's "alters" into one personality/identity.
   c. successful control of symptoms and distress caused by DID.
   d. successful recovery of memories that led to the client's disorder.

6. Which of the following is considered one of the most effective treatment strategies for the client who is engaged in individual therapy for a dissociative disorder?
   a. Supporting the client to talk about antecedent events around his or her feelings of anxiety and then planning behavioral technique to cope with stress
   b. Hypnosis for memory retrieval
   c. Amytal Sodium ("truth serum") interviews
   d. Use of SSRIs to reduce the client's defense mechanisms

7. Randi, age 20, has been admitted to the inpatient unit for DID. She just said, "I'm going to cut my wrist as soon as I can, with anything I can find on this unit!" Your most therapeutic nursing intervention would be:

a. "Randi, you need to calm down. Now, let's see if you have any prn medications ordered."

b. "That's not an option, Randi. You know we have removed all sharps from the area."

c. "Hold on, Randi. Let's go and talk about this before you go and do something that harmful to yourself."

d. "I understand that you are in pain right now. Let's take a minute to sit down and talk about how you're feeling."

8. In working with Randi, you are cautious about:

a. giving any medications, even if ordered as prn's.

b. using touch.

c. topics that Randi might want to talk about, especially self-mutilation.

d. engaging Randi's family in the treatment.

9. Goals for Randi while she is on the unit include all except which of the following?

a. Reduced verbalization about self-mutilation

b. Decreased episodes of dissociation

c. Refraining from acts of self-harm

d. Use of adaptive coping strategies and gaining of emotional control

10. Generalist nursing care of Randi will be focused on all except which of the following?

a. Educating her about the recovery process

b. Providing a safe and nonjudgmental environment

c. Helping her identify times when strong emotions can begin to overwhelm her

d. Facilitating Randi's alters to emerge and discuss their own perspectives

CHAPTER 22

The Client With a Personality Disorder

"Personality disorder" may be defined as a collection of personality characteristics that have become fixed and rigid to the point that the client experiences distress and behavioral dysfunction. Another definition refers to an enduring pattern of inner experience and behavior that deviates significantly from the expectations of the client's culture. Personality disorders can occur singularly or with other serious psychiatric disorders such as major depression, anxiety disorder, and substance abuse. The cause or causes of personality disorder are unknown. Determining an accurate prognosis for personality disorders is difficult. Based on reported clinical observations, some clients with personality disorders worsen over time, while others improve. Some clients drop out of treatment, preventing further follow-up; others refuse treatment, creating unknown variables in the study of this disorder.

Ten types of personality disorders are organized into three clusters: clusters A, B, and C. Clients with cluster A personality disorders typically are described as cold, withdrawn, suspicious, and irrational. Clients with cluster B personality disorders display dramatic, emotional, and attention-seeking behaviors. Clients with cluster C personality disorders often are anxious, tense, and over-controlled.

Clients with personality disorders may benefit from individual psychotherapy using supportive, insight-oriented, and cognitive-behavioral approaches. Group and family therapy may be beneficial for some clients with personality disorders.

Nurses require skill in assessing, forming trust, setting limits, and using therapeutic confrontation to provide effective care for clients with personality disorders. Nurses must be aware that progress in treating personality disorders usually is slow and requires patience and maturity on the part of the nurse and other treatment team members. For this reason, nurses must identify sources of personal and professional support to ensure their own health, survival, and growth.

LEARNING OBJECTIVES

After completing the exercises in this workbook, and studying the corresponding chapter in the textbook, the student will be able to:

- Define "personality disorder."
- Discuss the various etiological theories of the development of personality disorders.
- Explain the prognosis of personality disorders.
- Identify the types of personality disorders and their differentiating characteristics.
- Describe the treatment options available for clients with personality disorders.
- Apply the nursing process to the care of a person with personality disorder.

KEY TERMS

Personality: The totality of a person's unique biopsychosocial characteristics that consistently influences his or her inner experience and behavior across the lifespan.

Personality disorder: A collection of personality traits that have become fixed and rigid to the point that they impair the client's functioning and cause distress; also can be considered a lifelong pattern of behavior that affects many areas of the client's life, causes problems, and is not produced by another disorder or illness.

Splitting: Perceiving people and life experience in terms of "all good" or "all bad" categories.

Chapter Outline

PERSONALITY DISORDERS
Etiology
Signs and Symptoms/Diagnostic Criteria
Cluster A Personality Disorders
Paranoid Personality Disorder
Schizoid Personality Disorder
Schizotypal Personality Disorder
Cluster B Personality Disorders
Antisocial Personality Disorder
Borderline Personality Disorder
Histrionic Personality Disorder
Narcissistic Personality Disorder
Cluster C Personality Disorders
Avoidant Personality Disorder
Dependent Personality Disorder
Obsessive–Compulsive Personality Disorder

KEY TOPICS

Personality disorders: Cluster A (paranoid, schizoid, schizotypal); cluster B (antisocial, borderline, histrionic, narcissistic); cluster C (avoidant, dependent, obsessive–compulsive)

Interdisciplinary goals and treatment: Individual and group psychotherapies; family education and therapy

Nursing process: Assessment, diagnosis, planning, implementation (promoting participation in treatment; enlisting family; improving coping; reducing inappropriate behaviors; confronting; setting limits; providing for physical safety); evaluation

Nursing self-care

■ Exercises

There are many disorders of personality. Below are exercises designed to provide the student with an overview of each type, as well as exercises focusing on common goals and treatments for the personality clusters.

CASE STUDY EXERCISE

Here are three brief scenarios describing clients who have a specific personality disorder. After reviewing each, answer the questions below.

Bruce

Bruce, age 55, is single and lives with his parents, who are aging. He has worked for 35 years in a meat-packing plant, wrapping packages of meat for store deliveries. Bruce has no acquaintances or close friends and is described as a "loner." He rarely goes outside of his home, except to work and get groceries. When you speak with Bruce, he does not maintain eye contact; he speaks softly and taps his hands on the desk anxiously. He seems very reluctant to converse during your admission interview.

Roger

Roger, age 25, has been admitted to your unit for assessment following a fist fight that resulted in his breaking an arm and leg. Roger has been involved in numerous altercations, many of which have led him to serve brief periods of time in jail. He is often found in the community creating a disturbance of some sort, including drunken behavior, fighting, and shoplifting, for which he is often arrested. He is currently separated from his wife of 2 years. The separation, their first, occurred after he spanked their 2-year-old child, causing bruising on the child's buttocks. When you speak with Roger, he replies with short, clipped, and sarcastic answers. At one point, he jumps out of his chair, pretending to hit you with his casted right arm.

Gloria

Gloria, age 49, comes to the admission interview accompanied by Theodore, her husband of 32 years. Gloria is reluctant to speak with you at first, frequently looking down and glancing at Theodore. When she does speak, Gloria displays the language capability of an elementary school child and is unable to explain her feelings or thoughts about recent events. Several times during the interview, she turns to Theodore and makes statements such as: "Honey, why don't you tell her? You know I'm terrible at talking, and besides you know how I am better than I do."

1. Complete Table 22-1, using data from the vignettes, as well as information you know about signs and symptoms of these personality disorders.

TABLE 22–1. Vignette Questions

Add your hypothesis about which Personality Disorder is present, and in which Cluster it is found:	What are the signs and symptoms of this Personality Disorder (include those in the case study as well as others)?	Specific questions about this disorder:	Comment on any of the following for which you have data from the vignette:
Bruce: Cluster _____ Disorder:		How does Schizoid Personality differ from Schizophrenia?	Cognition: Affectivity: Behavior: Impulse Control:
Roger: Cluster _____ Disorder:		Why is Roger's disorder considered a Personality Disorder instead of "traits"?	Cognition: Affectivity: Behavior: Impulse Control:
Gloria: Cluster _____ Disorder:		What clues make you think Gloria has a Personality Disorder instead of just loving her husband very much?	Cognition: Affectivity: Behavior: Impulse Control:

2. Complete Table 22-2 by using data from Table 22-1 and interview data. Hypothesize about how each client might behave on a 22-bed inpatient psychiatric unit. For each of these clients, list selected nursing strategies you might use to intervene in three areas that are important for managing the inpatient unit milieu: limit-setting and confrontation about behaviors; safety issues; and participation in unit activities. Adapt your intervention style based on each client's particular personality characteristics. For example, because Bruce is withdrawn, you may want to encourage his active participation in all groups and activities, whereas with Roger you may need to limit the types and number of activities in which he is involved due to his lack of impulse control.

TABLE 22–2. Milieu Management Strategies for Personality Disordered Clients

Client	Milieu Management Strategies for Client Behaviors		
	Limit-Setting and Confrontation About Behaviors	Safety Issues	Participation in Unit Activities
Bruce			
Roger			
Gloria			

CRITICAL THINKING AND SELF-EVALUATION EXERCISES

1. Clients with personality disorders can often be difficult and challenging to work with. Nurses may experience fatigue, depression, and burnout when they are working with the client over time. Discuss ways that you can provide for self-care when working with clients with personality disorders.

2. Think about what might be the most challenging aspect of your work with clients with personality disorders. What type of personality disorder might you find most difficult to work with? Think about reasons why this may be true.

■ NCLEX-Style Exam Questions

1. The way in which personality disorders are different from personality traits is best described as follows:
   a. Disorders are usually evident earlier in the person's development than are traits.
   b. Traits usually cause the person a great deal of difficulty, but only sporadically.
   c. Disorders are usually more long-term than are traits.
   d. Disorders cause impairment in social and occupational functioning, whereas traits do not.

2. James has been suspicious of other clients on the unit, is often angry at others' comments, and carries a grudge against his roommate because the roommate accidentally used James' bath towel yesterday. Which of the following personality disorders is most likely James' diagnosis?
   a. Antisocial
   b. Paranoid
   c. Borderline
   d. Histrionic

3. Susan has been admitted to the inpatient unit for treatment of borderline personality disorder. Prior to admission, she was found in her parents' bedroom, burning her arm with an iron. This injury required a brief stay in the hospital's burn unit prior to transfer to your psychiatric unit. Which of the following is your highest nursing care priority, based on the above infor-

mation, for Susan during the first 24 hours of her admission?

a. Safety and protection from self-harm

b. Suicidal assessment

c. Working on Susan's self-esteem

d. Impulse control

4. Sheila, age 43, has been parading around the unit dressed in red high heels and a matching dress. She is seen sitting on the lap of a male client on the unit, and they are laughing. Which of the following is the most therapeutic nursing intervention?

a. "Sheila, you need to get off Tom's lap because that is inappropriate."

b. "Sheila, why are you sitting on Tom's lap?"

c. "Sheila, you need to go to your room because you are engaging in sexually provocative behavior again!"

d. "Sheila, why don't we go play a game of ping-pong?"

5. All except which of the following areas is identified in the *DSM-IV-TR* as one in which the majority of clients with personality disorders manifest symptoms?

a. Cognition

b. Affect

c. Impulse control

d. Suicidality

6. Behavior and characteristics of individuals with personality disorders are best described as

a. controlling.

b. provocative.

c. rigid and inflexible.

d. obnoxious and irritating.

7. Which of the following personality disorders is most often treated within the inpatient psychiatric setting?

a. Antisocial

b. Borderline

c. Schizotypal

d. Dependent

8. Which of the following nursing diagnoses would be least likely to be made when working with a client suffering from a personality disorder?

a. Ineffective Communication related to lack of orientation to reality

b. Noncompliance related to personality disorder

c. Ineffective Coping related to maladaptive personality traits

d. Risk for Suicide secondary to psychiatric illness

9. Cheryl has borderline personality disorder and lives at home with her parents. She has been in the psychiatric unit for 2 weeks and is scheduled to be discharged tomorrow. Which of the following would be most therapeutic when Cheryl's parents come in to discuss discharge plans?

a. Attempt to discuss placing Cheryl into an assisted living environment.

b. Ask the parents how they have coped with Cheryl's behaviors over the years.

c. Provide empathy to the parents, educate them about borderline personality disorder, and discuss their concerns about caring for Cheryl when she gets home.

d. Encourage the parents to discuss the possibility of Cheryl going into a day-care program when she goes home.

10. Cheryl asks you to go to lunch with her one day next week after her discharge. Your most therapeutic response to her request is:

a. "That sounds good. Call the unit when you decide which day, and we can set it up."

b. "Cheryl, I'd love to do that, but I'm on vacation next week."

c. "Going out to lunch would not be appropriate, because you are the patient and I'm your nurse. I'm sorry, but I can't work with you after discharge."

d. "Cheryl, that is not possible. Let's discuss why you feel you would like to do that."

CHAPTER 23

The Client With an Eating Disorder

Anorexia nervosa and bulimia nervosa primarily affect young women. Anorexia nervosa and bulimia nervosa share many etiologic factors and may be viewed as existing along a single spectrum of eating disorders. Although multiple theories exist, most experts agree that eating disorders develop from a complex interaction of individual, family, and sociocultural factors. Clients with eating disorders exhibit disturbances in many or all the functional health patterns.

Treatment of clients with eating disorders occurs in community-based and inpatient settings and is a complex and often lengthy process. In the current climate of healthcare reform, short-term therapies such as CBT, IPT, and SFBT are increasingly used. Desired client outcomes include normalization of weight and eating patterns, improved self-esteem, and development of realistic thought processes, adaptive coping mechanisms, and constructive family processes. Most clients require follow-up treatment to reinforce behavioral changes and prevent a return of disordered eating.

LEARNING OBJECTIVES

After completing the exercises in this workbook, and studying the corresponding chapter in the textbook, the student will be able to:

- Describe the incidence of eating disorders and the populations most commonly affected by them.

- Discuss possible etiologies of eating disorders.

- Distinguish between anorexia nervosa and bulimia nervosa.

- Describe the *DSM-IV-TR* diagnostic criteria for anorexia nervosa and bulimia nervosa.

- Describe interdisciplinary goals and treatment of clients with eating disorders.

- Apply the nursing process to the care of clients with eating disorders.

KEY TERMS

Amenorrhea: Absence of or abnormal cessation of menstruation.

Anorexia nervosa: A life-threatening eating disorder characterized by disturbed body image, emaciation, and intense fear of becoming obese.

Binge eating: Uncontrollable consumption of large amounts of food.

Binge eating disorder: An eating disorder characterized by recurrent episodes of binge eating, with accompanying marked distress and impaired control over such behavior.

Bulimia nervosa: An eating disorder characterized by binge eating, followed by purging.

Emotional reasoning: A cognitive distortion by which a person relies on his or her subjective emotions to determine reality.

Purging: Attempting to eliminate the body of excess calories; examples of purging methods include self-induced vomiting, use of laxatives, and excessive exercise.

Chapter Outline

EATING DISORDERS
Etiology
Biologic Theories
Behavioral Theories
Sociocultural Theories
Family-Based Theories
Signs and Symptoms/Diagnostic Criteria
Anorexia Nervosa
Bulimia Nervosa
Comorbidities and Dual Diagnoses
Implications and Prognosis
Interdisciplinary Goals and Treatment
Behavioral Therapy
Cognitive Therapy
Cognitive-Behavioral Therapy
Interpersonal Therapy
Solution-Focused Brief Therapy
Family Therapy
Group Therapy

Pharmacologic Interventions
APPLICATION OF THE NURSING PROCESS TO CLIENTS WITH EATING DISORDERS
Assessment
History and Physical Examination
Psychosocial Assessment
Nursing Diagnosis
Planning
Implementation
Restoring Nutritional Balance
Encouraging Realistic Thinking Processes
Improving Body Image
Building Self-Esteem
Exploring Feelings of Powerlessness
Encouraging Effective Coping
Restoring Family Processes
  Enmeshment and Overprotectiveness
  Conflict Avoidance and Rigidity
Evaluation

KEY TOPICS

Eating disorders: Etiology (biologic, behavioral, socio-cultural, family theories)

Signs and symptoms: Anorexia nervosa; bulimia nervosa

Interdisciplinary goals and treatment: Therapies (behavioral, cognitive; cognitive-behavioral; interpersonal; solution-focused brief; family; group); pharmacology

Nursing process: Assessment; diagnosis; planning; implementation (nutrition; realistic thinking; body image and self-esteem; powerlessness; coping; family processes); evaluation

■ Exercises

CASE STUDY EXERCISE

Rose P., age 23, has been admitted to your unit with a diagnosis of bulimia nervosa after a suicide attempt by using alcohol and Tylenol. She was found in her bedroom by a friend. On the admission interview, Rose states, "Since I was 20, I have had this problem of eating huge amounts of food in one sitting, and then vomiting. In fact, I think there is rarely a time when I eat and don't vomit afterwards. I think people are beginning to notice that I immediately go to the bathroom after I eat."

1. What is the first nursing care priority for Rose during her first 24 hours on the unit?

2. Using your textbook Table 23-1, describe how you would assess Rose's functional health patterns. Provide questions that are specific to Rose.

You have determined that Rose is no longer suicidal, and you begin to focus on her eating disorder. From the functional health patterns, you discover that Rose binges and purges at least once a day, and this has been going on for about 2 months. Prior to that, she had been doing this behavior two or three times per week. She reports, "I just can't help it; there's nothing I have tried that can stop me from doing this, and it's really upsetting." Additionally, she says, "I also sometimes use a laxative just to help clear out my intestines." She believes that her friends think she is extremely overweight, although she cannot state exactly what they have said that would lead her to believe this.

3. Explain, in as much detail as possible, the neuro-chemical disturbances that are believed to be occurring in Rose's case, including neurobiology and neuroendocrine systems.

4. Does genetics play a role in bulimia nervosa? What is the current evidence for this?

5. What medications have been suggested for treating bulimia nervosa? Include any teaching you would need to do with Rose if she were placed on one of these medications.

After Rose has been on the unit for 2 days, she begins to talk with you about some of her thoughts and feelings about her condition. She states, "Since I've been here, I think I am gaining weight. Yesterday in group, everyone said that I was 'looking better,' and I think they can all tell I've gained 4 pounds since admission." When you begin to work with Rose on this cognitive distortion, she states, "I know what you mean. I probably am overinterpreting what they said in group, but I know that they see me as a fat person. My parents do, too. When I binge, it just feels like I might as well go ahead and eat the whole gallon of ice cream, because my figure is already totally ruined." Further problem solving with Rose leads to a discussion about life in general. She says, "I have never been able to find a guy who will date me, and I know full well it's related to my heavy weight. I mean, I look around here and see other clients being visited by their husbands and boyfriends, and they have such ideal lives. I think if I could just tackle this problem, my life would be so perfect; I'm basically very happy with the rest of my life."

6. From the above data and textbook Table 23-2, identify three cognitive distortions manifested by Rose. Name each distortion, explain what about it is distorted, and briefly discuss how you might respond to each statement in a therapeutic manner.

7. Complete the Nursing Process Worksheet on the next page, focusing on cognitive distortions as a nursing diagnosis. Describe interventions that may be useful in helping Rose to reduce these distortions.

8. Rose's parents and her 20-year-old sister come in for a family meeting. Her parents and sister state that they are very supportive of Rose's efforts to get better, and they want to learn how to help in this process. What suggestions can you offer to the family to help them accomplish this?

CRITICAL THINKING AND SELF-EVALUATION EXERCISE

1. Think about how eating disorders are perceived on your campus. Do you know anyone with an eating disorder? Is treatment available on your campus for students who may be suffering from an eating disorder?

■ NCLEX-Style Exam Questions

1. Studies from the NIMH suggest that eating disorders may be associated with excessive levels of which brain hormone?
   a. Vasopressin
   b. Dopamine
   c. Prolactin
   d. Neuropeptide P

2. Debbie is 5-foot-6, weighs 105 lb, exercises 4 hours per day, and does not engage in any binging or purging behaviors. She believes that she is becoming obese and states, "I'm shocked that you think I'm underweight. You don't understand me." Debbie's most likely diagnosis is
   a. anorexia nervosa, binge eating and purging type.

   b. bulimia nervosa, nonpurging type.
   c. anorexia nervosa, restricting type.
   d. eating disorder not otherwise specified.

3. Debbie's laboratory results will likely be abnormal in all except which of the following ways?
   a. Increased serum cholesterol
   b. Increased BUN
   c. Normal serum albumin
   d. Low cortisol levels

4. Susan's dentist noticed that her teeth were losing enamel. When asked about this, Susan states that this "runs in her family." Which of the eating disorders is most often associated with dental carries and enamel loss?
   a. Bulimia nervosa, purging type
   b. Anorexia nervosa, restricting type
   c. Eating disorder not otherwise specified
   d. Bulimia nervosa, nonpurging type

5. Behavior family systems therapy (BFST) is often used with clients who have anorexia nervosa. This approach to treatment includes four phases
   a. weight gain, cognitive restructuring, weight maintenance, discharge.
   b. assessment, control rationale, weight gain, and weight maintenance.
   c. assessment, planning, intervention, and evaluation.
   d. weight gain, assessment, control rationale, and evaluation.

6. Which of the following medications has been found to be worthy of a trial in clients with bulimia nervosa who have obsessive–compulsive traits?
   a. Prozac (fluoxetine)
   b. Lithium
   c. Haloperidol (Haldol)
   d. Bupropion (BuSpar)

7. All except which of the following are likely findings on physical examination of the client with anorexia nervosa?
   a. Dehydration
   b. Lanugo
   c. Amenorrhea
   d. Hyperkalemia

NURSING PROCESS WORKSHEET

Health Problem (Title)

Client Goal*

Related to

↓

Etiology (Related Factors)

Nursing Interventions**

Evidenced by

↓

**Signs and Symptoms
(Defining Characteristics)**

Evaluative Statement

*More than one client goal may be appropriate. For this exercise, choose one client goal that demonstrates a direct resolution of the client problem identified in the nursing diagnosis.

**Be sure you are able to list the scientific rationale for each nursing intervention you order.

8. When admitted to the inpatient unit, Joyce is 5-foot-10 and weighs 100 lb. What is the initial goal in her care?

    a. To stop losing weight

    b. To be on bedrest

    c. To reduce her fluid intake

    d. To assess for violence potential

9. Many clients with eating disorders suffer from distortions in thinking. Personalization involves which of the following?

    a. Giving an event or its consequences more merit than is realistic

    b. Reasoning by extremes

    c. Overgeneralizing beliefs on one or a few considerations

    d. Overinterpreting an event as having personal significance

10. Shana, who has anorexia and weighs less than 85% of her normal body weight, says, "I'm so fat, I can't even get through this doorway, much less fit into any of my clothes." Your most therapeutic response is

    a. "Shana, let's talk about your ideas about your body and why you perceive yourself to be fat."

    b. "Shana, you must try and stop thinking that way. Let's think of some alternative ideas for describing your body."

    c. "Shana, you only weigh 100 lb. It is just not true that you are fat."

    d. "Shana, I understand what you are saying. However, you are under your ideal body weight, and it is causing you to have the medical problems that we have talked about."

CHAPTER 24

The Client With a Mood Disorder

Mood disorders include major depressive disorder, dysthymic disorder, and bipolar disorder. Mood disorders are a significant problem in America, and suicide, which is closely associated with mood disorders, is an emergent national public health priority. The etiology of mood disorders is complex and involves multiple interactions between genetic factors, physiological factors, and psychological factors. Signs and symptoms and diagnostic criteria for the mood disorders are categorized by diagnosis and are highly specific.

Mood disorders are often unrecognized and go untreated; however, when clients receive appropriate treatment, the mood disorders are highly treatable, with good outcomes. There are multiple treatment modalities for clients with mood disorders, including individual, group, and family psychotherapies, pharmacotherapy, and somatic therapies.

Psychiatric–mental health nurses must use the nursing process to assess, plan, implement, and evaluate care for individuals who have mood disorders. Nursing assessment is the first step of the nursing process and involves systematic, thorough consideration of the client's safety, psychological functioning or mental status, physiological and psychomotor activity, and social and behavioral functioning. From data gathered during the assessment process, the nurse identifies the client's potential or actual problems in functioning, formulates nursing diagnoses, and specifies client behavior outcomes that guide the planning of interventions. Following intervention, the nurse evaluates the effectiveness of the interventions in contributing to desired outcomes, makes changes and improvements, and continues through with the assessment process.

LEARNING OBJECTIVES

After completing the exercises in this workbook, and studying the corresponding chapter in the textbook, the student will be able to:

- Describe examples of mood disorders.

- Discuss the incidence and prevalence of major mood disorders in the United States.

- Analyze differences between theories of the etiology of mood disorders.

- List the symptoms of depressive and bipolar disorders using *DSM-IV-TR* criteria.

- Discuss interdisciplinary treatment modalities for clients with mood disorders.

- Apply the nursing process to the care of clients with mood disorders.

KEY TERMS

Affect: The outward expression of emotion; it is of shorter duration, more variable, and more reactive than underlying mood, which is more pervasive and stable.

Cyclothymia: A disorder resembling bipolar disorder but with less severe symptoms, characterized by repeated periods of nonpsychotic depression and hypomania for at least 2 years (1 year for children and adolescents).

Dysthymia: A milder form of depressive illness in which symptoms are less severe than in depressive disorder, but may be chronic.

Electroconvulsive therapy (ECT): A therapy that involves the application of a small dose of electricity to one or both sides of the brain to induce a seizure.

Hypomania: A subcategory of mania, slightly less severe and without the psychotic features or severely impaired functioning that would require hospitalization.

Manic episodes: Periods of abnormally and persistently elevated, expansive, or irritable mood.

Mood: A pervasive, sustained emotional coloring of one's experience.

Phototherapy: Use of artificial light therapy to prevent and treat depression with a seasonal pattern.

Chapter Outline

KEY TOPICS

Mood disorders etiology: Genetic factors; physiological factors (biogenic amines [norepinephrine, dopamine, serotonin]; psychoneuroendocrinology); psychological factors (psychodynamic factors, learned helplessness, cognitive, feminist)

Signs and symptoms/diagnostic criteria: Major depressive disorder; dysthymic disorder; bipolar disorders (bipolar I and II; cyclothymic)

Interdisciplinary goals and treatment: Psychotherapy; cognitive-behavioral therapy; pharmacological therapies; somatic nonpharmacological therapies

Nursing process: Assessment (safety, mental status examination, physiological stability, family issues); diagnosis; planning; implementation (protecting client from suicide; potential for violence; physical health; thought processes); evaluation

■ Exercises

CASE STUDY EXERCISE

Randy K., age 18, is a high school student who was admitted to the acute psychiatric unit following an attempted suicide. Randy had come home from school early and hanged himself in his bedroom on the closet clothes rod. His father happened to get off work that day at 3:30, arriving just in time to get Randy down from the closet and dial 911. Randy barely escaped death, is medically stable, and has been transferred from the emergency department to your psychiatric unit. Randy's parents report that over the past 6 months, they have noticed a decline in his functioning in school, making C's when he used to be a straight B student. He has become more withdrawn, often spending most of his time at home in his bedroom. He has lost 25 lb in the past 6 months, has complained of fatigue, and has even converted his entire wardrobe to black clothing. His parents state that they have been "worried about Randy, but we just didn't know what we should do, and we thought it was normal teenager behavior." They describe their son as a stable, responsible, "well-balanced" child who has always brought them pride. He has never been impulsive or done any of the "typical teenage things, like smoking, drugging, or drinking," so they were "really shocked that he's so depressed."

During the week prior to his suicide attempt, Randy said, he had been "staying awake all night and trying to sleep during the day. I skipped 4 days of school last week because I just couldn't concentrate. I haven't eaten anything in about 3 days and I'm not even hungry. I know I'm a bad son and that I just can't live up to my parents' expectations of me." He also says that he has been thinking about death a lot since last semester, when one of his classmates died in an auto accident. He says he didn't really know the student that well, but when the accident happened, it made him start thinking "about how fragile life is, and that you just never know when your time is going to be up."

1. Using Box 24-7 in Textbook Chapter 24 list questions you need to ask of Randy to complete a comprehensive assessment of his suicidality. Discuss data that you have from the above, and identify what data you still need to obtain.

2. Discuss other elements that need to be addressed in a comprehensive nursing admission assessment of Randy.

3. "Potential for self-harm" is the critical nursing concern for Randy's first 24 hours after admission. Using the Nursing Process Worksheet on the next page, outline a comprehensive nursing care plan for keeping Randy safe on the unit.

On the second day of hospitalization, Randy is started on Prozac, 20 mg/day. He has remained suicidal and has been on suicide precautions since admission. He is remaining in his room most of the day, but does come out to eat meals in the dining room.

4. Explain the mechanism of action of Prozac (ie, how does it act at the synapse?). Also list the category of drug, side effects, and dosage range. Is this an appropriate dose for Randy?

5. Describe what you will need to teach Randy about his new medication.

6. A rare side effect of Prozac is serotonin syndrome. Discuss the symptoms of serotonin syndrome; describe why it would be important to recognize this syndrome in a client.

During a family meeting, you discover that Randy's uncle (his mother's brother) committed suicide when the uncle was 23 years old. Randy's mother reports that since Randy's admission, she has been having difficulty sleeping and eating and has been crying almost every day. She states, "I just was so upset when John committed suicide, because I was only 16 years old at that time. I'm so afraid that Randy has the same thing John did, but we never really knew why John did it. He had not had any problems before he did it."

7. Using Table 24-1 in Textbook Chapter 24 discuss how might you intervene with Mrs. K during the family meeting.

8. How might you help the family deal with Randy's recent attempt? Where could you refer them (especially Mrs. K.) for additional help?

After 2 weeks on Prozac, Randy's depression has lifted. He is social in the unit and has been relating in a humorous way with the other clients. He has begun to eat three meals a day and to sleep through the night. When you ask about his feelings, he states, "I can't believe how good I feel. I didn't realize how depressed I was. I just feel that my life is wide open now, and I can really do anything I want to with my life. I just don't feel sad at all."

9. Two to three weeks after beginning an antidepressant is a period of risk for the suicidal client. Discuss why this is so.

10. What nursing interventions can you implement that will reduce Randy's risk for a suicide attempt during this critical period of recovery?

CRITICAL THINKING AND SELF-EVALUATION EXERCISES

1. What are your thoughts about people who contemplate suicide? Prior to reading the textbook chapter on depression, what were your ideas about why people might think about suicide? Have your ideas changed?

NURSING PROCESS WORKSHEET

Health Problem (Title)	Client Goal*
Related to ↓	
Etiology (Related Factors)	Nursing Interventions**
Evidenced by ↓	
Signs and Symptoms (Defining Characteristics)	Evaluative Statement

*More than one client goal may be appropriate. For this exercise, choose one client goal that demonstrates a direct resolution of the client problem identified in the nursing diagnosis.

**Be sure you are able to list the scientific rationale for each nursing intervention you order.

2. If you were caring for a client who was suicidal, what might be some of your concerns related to your own professional role?

■ NCLEX-Style Exam Questions

1. In regard to genetic transmission of bipolar disorders, which of the following is true?
   a. The mode of transmission is very complex but seems to involve susceptibility loci on chromosomal regions 18p, 18q, and 21q.
   b. Bipolar disorders show no evidence of genetic transmission.
   c. Bipolar disorder has been shown to be a defect on chromosome 22.
   d. Bipolar disorders have not been seen to cross generational boundaries.

2. The monoamine hypothesis of depression
   a. holds that depression is caused by sociocultural and psychological factors.
   b. holds that depression is caused by only one of the biogenic amines
   c. holds that depression results from a deficiency in the concentrations or in metabolic dysregulation of the monoamines.
   d. relates to bipolar disorders, not to depression.

3. When an individual is subjected to chronic, uncontrollable stress, which of the following is most accurate?
   a. Hypoactivity of the HPA results, which leads to depression.
   b. The HPA axis becomes inactive, causing the brain to overproduce monoamine neurotransmitters.
   c. Hyperactivity of the HPA results, which leads to hypersecretion of adrenal glucocorticoids and CRF, both of which contribute to mood disorders.
   d. The individual makes physical and psychological responses to the stress that immediately attenuate the stress response.

4. Susan was abandoned by her parents at age 3, resulting in her perception of the world as a hostile place and the subsequent development of rage against men. This statement is an example of

   a. why Susan has become lesbian at the age of 23.
   b. a psychodynamic interpretation of Susan's major depressive disorder.
   c. a biophysiological explanation for Susan's depressive disorder.
   d. a feminist viewpoint of depression.

5. The following statement, "People who are susceptible to mood disorders have encountered a lifetime of experiences that have taught them that they are ineffective and have no influence on the factors that cause their suffering," captures the major ideas behind
   a. Freud's theory of depression.
   b. Seligman's learned helplessness model.
   c. Beck's cognitive triad of depression.
   d. Adler's theory of psychoneuroimmunology.

6. The major difference between bipolar I and bipolar II disorder is that
   a. clients with bipolar I have no symptoms of mania, but only depression.
   b. the prognosis for bipolar I is much better than for bipolar II.
   c. both disorders are the same, except that clients with bipolar I disorders have a much higher incidence of suicide.
   d. clients with bipolar II disorder do not have symptoms of mania that interfere enough to cause marked functional disturbances.

7. James T. is admitted to the unit in an acute manic episode. He has had three major depressive episodes in the past 10 years and two other hospitalizations for mania. Which of the following disorders would reflect James' symptom profile?
   a. Bipolar I
   b. Bipolar II
   c. Cyclothymic disorder
   d. Dysthymic disorder

8. James is running up and down the hallway without a shirt or shoes. He is entering other clients' rooms and singing to them. What is the most appropriate nursing intervention?
   a. "James, you need to calm down and walk with me to get some medications that will help you."

b. "James, you need to come with me to your room to get clothing. If you cannot keep yourself in the dining area, you will need to stay in your room for a while."

c. "James, it's not okay to sing on the unit. You are upsetting everyone else."

d. "James, why are you running, and where is your shirt?"

9. James has been on lithium, 300 mg qid, for 3 weeks now. He approaches you, saying, "I feel like I'm going to toss my cookies, and I can't even hold this cup of coffee straight. Why can't I do the crossword puzzle? I usually can do them in about 5 minutes." What is the appropriate nursing intervention at this time?

a. Further assess James' symptoms, call the MD, hold his next dose of lithium, and have a blood level drawn because he is evidencing symptoms of toxicity.

b. Explain to James that these are normal side effects of the lithium, and he will get accustomed to them over time.

c. Try to refocus James onto another task, because his mania is causing him to be agitated.

d. Talk with a colleague about James' symptoms, and get assistance in deciding what to do next.

10. Carrie, age 20, was admitted to your unit following a lethal suicide attempt. She is disheveled, disorganized, and dehydrated. The priority for her care during the first 24 hours of her admission is:

a. rehydrating Carrie by forcing fluids.

b. assisting Carrie with her activities of daily living, including a shower and clean clothing.

c. assessing Carrie's recent suicide attempt, and identifying factors that may have contributed to it.

d. assessing Carrie's current suicidal ideation, and putting Carrie on suicide precautions.

CHAPTER 25

The Client With a Thought Disorder

This chapter focuses on schizophrenia, the most common and severe psychotic disorder, affecting 1% of the population. Other psychotic disorders include schizophreniform disorder, schizoaffective disorder, delusional disorder, brief psychotic disorder, shared psychotic disorder, and psychosis not otherwise specified. Schizophrenia is most likely not a single disease of the brain but a heterogeneous disorder with some common features, including thought disturbances and preoccupation with frightening inner experiences and disturbances of affect, behavior, and socialization. The major theories of etiology are biological, including genetic, neurochemical and neuropathological, viral, immunological, and structural abnormalities. There are five subtypes of schizophrenia: paranoid, disorganized, catatonic, undifferentiated, and residual.

Antipsychotic medications are the primary treatment for a client with schizophrenia. There are two types of antipsychotics: traditional and atypical. Traditional antipsychotics primarily treat the positive symptoms of schizophrenia and are associated with numerous and distressing extrapyramidal side effects. The atypical antipsychotics treat both the positive and negative symptoms of schizophrenia and typically cause fewer side effects.

Continuity of care for the schizophrenic client is essential. It involves discharge planning and aggressive care within the community setting. Nursing intervention for the client with schizophrenia focuses on safety, acceptance, medication education and adherence, intervening in hallucinations and delusions, social skills, self-care, and education.

LEARNING OBJECTIVES

After completing the exercises in this workbook, and studying the corresponding chapter in the textbook, the student will be able to:

- Define "schizophrenia."

- Compare other thought disorders with schizophrenia.

- Discuss the proposed etiologies of schizophrenia.

- Identify signs and symptoms of schizophrenia.

- Describe the subtypes of schizophrenia.

- Compare the benefits versus risks of antipsychotic medications.

- Explain the continuum of care for people with schizophrenia.

- Apply the nursing process to the care of a person with schizophrenia.

- Identify self-care for nurses working with clients with schizophrenia.

KEY TERMS

Affect: An observable behavior that expresses feeling or emotional tone; it refers to more fluctuating changes in emotional "weather."

Affective flattening/blunting: A reduced intensity of emotional expression and response.

Alogia: A poverty of thinking that is inferred from observing the client's language and speech.

Anhedonia: The loss of capacity to experience pleasure subjectively.

Apathy: The seeming absence of caring about self or others.

Avolition: The inability to start, persist in, and carry through to its logical conclusion any goal-directed activity.

Delusions: Fixed, false beliefs about external reality that reasoning cannot correct; these include but are not limited to the following types: grandiose (beliefs involving inflated self-worth, power, or knowledge); persecutory (belief that one is being attacked, harassed, cheated, or conspired against); and somatic (beliefs that give false attributions to the appearance or functioning of one's body).

Dual diagnosis: Diagnosis of a serious mental illness in addition to a substance abuse disorder or an addiction to a substance.

Extrapyramidal side effects (EPS): The most common and distressing side effects associated with traditional antipsychotic medications; they include akathisia (severe restlessness), dystonia (muscle spasm or contraction), chronic motor problems such as tardive dyskinesia, and the pseudoparkinsonian symptoms of rigidity, mask-like facies, and stiff gait.

Hallucination: Sensory perception with a compelling sense of reality; types include auditory (involving the perception of sound); gustatory (involving the perception of taste); olfactory (involving the perception of odor); tactile (involving the perception of being touched or of something under the skin); visual (involving sight, such as seeing images, people, flashes of light); and somatic (involving perception of a physical experience localized within the body).

Mood: A sustained emotional "climate."

Schizophrenia: A heterogeneous disorder of the brain with features including thought disturbances and pre-occupation with frightening inner experiences (eg, delusions and hallucinations), affect disturbances (eg, flat or inappropriate affect), and behavioral/social disturbances (eg, unpredictable, bizarre behavior or social isolation).

Tardive dyskinesia (TD): An extrapyramidal symptom characterized by abnormal, involuntary, and irregular choreoathetoid (writhing) movements, most predominantly in the head and facial region.

Thought disorders: Serious and often persistent mental illnesses characterized by disturbances in reality orientation, thinking, and social involvement.

Vulnerability model (stress-vulnerability model): Psychosocial theory that states that schizophrenia is characterized by vulnerability rather than continuous symptoms.

Water intoxication: A problem that sometimes accompanies schizophrenia in which a client drinks excessive water, thereby developing polyuria and hyponatremia; when severe enough, this condition can result in seizures, coma, cerebral edema, and even death.

Chapter Outline

SCHIZOPHRENIA AND OTHER THOUGHT DISORDERS
The Stigma of Schizophrenia
Etiology
Biological Theories
  Genetic Influences
  Neurochemical and Neuroanatomical Changes
Psychosocial Theories
Signs and Symptoms/Diagnostic Criteria
The Disorganization Dimension
  Disorganized Speech
  Disorganized Behavior
  Incongruous Affect
The Psychotic Dimension
  Delusions

  Hallucinations
The Negative Dimension
Other Symptoms
Subtypes of Schizophrenia
Water Intoxication in Schizophrenia
Comorbidities and Dual Diagnoses
Implications and Prognosis
Interdisciplinary Goals and Treatment
Pharmacological Interventions
  Traditional (Conventional) Antipsychotics
  Atypical (Novel) Antipsychotics
Psychosocial Interventions
  Milieu Management
  Individual and Group Therapy
  Cognitive-behavioral Therapy
  Vocational Rehabilitation
Continuum of Care
  Discharge Planning
  Care in the Community
    Assertive Community Treatment (ACT)
    Intensive Case Management (ICM)
APPLICATION OF THE NURSING PROCESS TO THE CLIENT WITH A THOUGHT DISORDER
Assessment
Assessing Mood and Cognitive State
Assessing Potential for Violence
Assessing Social Support
Assessing Knowledge
Nursing Diagnosis
Planning
Implementation
Intervening in Disturbed Thought Processes and Sensory Perceptions
  Reinforcing Reality
  Understanding Language Content
  Intervening in Hallucinations
Managing Violent Behavior
Lessening Social Isolation
  Developing Trust
  Initiating Interaction
  Modeling Affect
Promoting Adherence to Medication Regimens
Promoting Improved Individual Coping Skills
Strengthening Family Processes
Providing Client and Family Education
  Teaching Symptom Management
Evaluation

KEY TOPICS

Schizophrenia and other thought disorders: Stigma; etiologies; signs and symptoms; comorbidities and dual diagnosis; implications and prognosis

Interdisciplinary goals and treatment: Pharmacological and psychosocial interventions; the continuum of care

The nursing process: Assessment, diagnosis, planning and intervention (managing violent behavior, reducing isolation, strengthening individual and family coping, client and family education, symptom management)

■ Exercises

CASE STUDY EXERCISE

Joe J., age 22, has been admitted to the inpatient unit with chronic schizophrenia, paranoid type. When you approach Joe for the initial admission assessment, he is in his room, lying in bed with the covers over his head. When you say hello, he replies, "I don't want to be here, because everyone is trying to hurt me. I am going to stay in my bed, so don't even try to get me out."

1. List two possible approaches to Joe at this time, and give your rationale for each. One example is provided.

   a. Possible Response (example): *"Joe, I would like to spend a little time with you to talk about how you are doing right now. I know this must be difficult for you."*

      Rationale: *Joe is frightened and anxious about being in a new and unfamiliar place. Engaging him by stating what your purpose is and reflecting empathy is a way to build trust. Because he is paranoid, trust is a major issue for Joe.*

   b. Possible Response: _____
      _____
      _____
      _____

      Rationale: _____
      _____
      _____
      _____
      _____

   c. Possible Response: _____
      _____
      _____
      _____
      _____

Rationale: _____
_____
_____
_____
_____
_____

When you respond to Joe, he comes out from under the covers and sits on the edge of his bed. His eyes are darting around and he appears anxious. He remains on the edge of the bed as you sit down in the chair at his desk in the room. You begin to ask Joe some questions about how he came to the hospital, and he tells you that he was living at home with his parents and had begun to stay in his bedroom all day. He says, "I don't know why they wouldn't leave me alone. All I wanted was some quiet." Joe asks you how many people work here and how many people are on the unit. He states that he believes he is being filmed and asks, "How long will I have to stay here?"

2. From the data presented thus far in the case study, list the symptoms that lead you to believe Joe is suffering from schizophrenia.

3. What do you think is Joe's underlying concern in asking questions about length of hospitalization?

4. Provide at least two therapeutic responses to Joe's questions at this point:

   a. _____
      _____
      _____

   b. _____
      _____
      _____

In reviewing Joe's medical record, you see that Joe has been on several antipsychotic medications since he was diagnosed at age 19. He tends to have paranoid ideation, with hallucinations and delusions when he is most ill. However, his history shows that once on medications, he stabilizes quickly and has been able to maintain his grades in a local community college. The medications he has been on recently (including Haldol, Mellaril, and a trial of loxapine) are described by him as follows: "I get totally snowed. They make me so groggy, I can't keep up with my homework. So I've been just stopping them, because school is very important to me."

5. Explain why these medications are making Joe so groggy, including their general mechanisms of action, and why they would cause drowsiness.

6. Which neurotransmitters are targeted by these medications?

7. What other antipsychotic medications may be more helpful for Joe's symptoms? Why might they be more effective than the ones he has tried?

While on the unit, Joe has difficulty getting up in the morning. He sleeps until 11 a.m. or noon and spends most of the afternoon in his room reading. His hygiene is poor, with infrequent showers and clothing that smells. When you talk with Joe about this, he becomes agitated, stating, "I'll dress the way I want and get up when I want. You can't tell me what to do." You acknowledge that these are choices Joe has the ability to make.

Later that day, you talk with Joe about his behaviors again and ask whether they get in the way of his going to school when he is at home. Joe says it is a problem for him when he is trying to attend school and cannot get up in the morning and take care of himself, but he states that he has given up trying to "fix this problem" because it seems too difficult. You tell Joe that perhaps together you and he can develop some goals and find a way to meet them. He is willing to work with you because school is an important part of his life, and he needs to be able to attend.

8. Complete the Nursing Process Worksheet on the following page. Develop two nursing diagnoses around Joe's problems with hygiene and daily activities; set several goals for Joe, nursing interventions, and evaluative criteria.

Joe is placed on a trial of Clozaril, 300 mg, b.i.d. He has not been on this medication before.

9. What type of medication is Clozaril? Explain the drug's mechanism of action and major side effects.

10. Which of Joe's symptoms do you predict will be most affected by Clozaril? Why?

11. Develop a brief teaching plan for Joe, explaining the target symptoms, side effects, and important things to watch for when he is on this medication.

12. What follow-up is needed, if any, after Joe is placed on Clozaril?

Joe is being discharged to home after a 3-week hospitalization. His symptoms have stabilized, and he reports, "I feel better than I have in quite a while. I think this medication is really helping me."

13. List at least two issues that need to be addressed in Joe's discharge planning. What is the nurse's role in ensuring that each of these issues is dealt with before he leaves the hospital?

a. Issue: _____

Nurse's Role: _____

_____

b. Issue: _____

Nurse's Role: _____

_____

CRITICAL THINKING AND SELF-EVALUATION EXERCISES

1. Have you ever known anyone who has schizophrenia? If so, what types of symptoms did you observe? How did the illness affect you?

2. Imagine what it would be like to feel that everyone in your life was against you and wanted to hurt you. Identify and discuss some of the feelings that you might experience.

■ NCLEX-Style Exam Questions

1. All except which of the following have been proposed as potential mechanisms for the etiology of thought disorders?

   a. Inadequate mothering during critical developmental periods
   b. Genetic predispositions
   c. Dysregulation of neurotransmitter systems
   d. Hemispheric brain dysfunction

NURSING PROCESS WORKSHEET

Health Problem (Title)

Client Goal*

Related to

↓

Etiology (Related Factors)

Nursing Interventions**

Evidenced by

↓

**Signs and Symptoms
(Defining Characteristics)**

Evaluative Statement

*More than one client goal may be appropriate. For this exercise, choose one client goal that demonstrates a direct resolution of the client problem identified in the nursing diagnosis.
**Be sure you are able to list the scientific rationale for each nursing intervention you order.

2. John comes into the emergency department stating, "I'm scared because the FBI is now tapping my home phone, and I can hear them talking between my two telephones during the night." John appears disheveled, smells of urine, and speaks in broken sentences. His eyes dart around the room while you are trying to interview him, and he is tapping his fingers on the table. Your first nursing priority with John would be to

   a. assess his family for dysfunctional dynamics.

   b. reassure John that he is in a safe place where he will be helped.

   c. speak with John about calling members of his family to come in.

   d. give John Haldol IM to reduce his paranoia.

3. Sarah states, "My boss keeps putting thoughts into my head. Yesterday she made me copy 25 reports and then told me I had wasted company time and money!" Sarah is experiencing

   a. thought withdrawal.

   b. thought blocking.

   c. thought insertion.

   d. thought broadcasting.

4. Steven had been withdrawn in his room for 3 days, not eating or sleeping, prior to his admission to your inpatient unit. When you interview him on intake, Steven demonstrates difficulty answering questions, appears to have no facial expressions, and cannot follow simple instructions. Together, these symptoms are commonly referred to as

   a. delusions.

   b. thought disorder.

   c. negative symptoms.

   d. positive symptoms.

5. Yolanda has been on Haldol for 5 years. When she is admitted to the inpatient unit for a recent exacerbation of her schizophrenic symptoms, you assess that she has akathisia, dystonia, a stiff gait, and rigid posture. You realize that these are symptoms of

   a. psychosis.

   b. tardive dyskinesia.

   c. extrapyramidal side effects of Haldol.

   d. the normal process of schizophrenia over time.

6. When you consider interventions for Yolanda's symptoms, the following would be most appropriate:

   a. Let her symptoms go, because they are normal and can't be changed.

   b. Give her Navane instead of Haldol.

   c. Consult with the psychiatrist and suggest that she be placed on an anticholinergic drug.

   d. Remove the Haldol to see whether it is the reason for these symptoms.

7. The major difference between the typical and atypical antipsychotics is that

   a. typical antipsychotics most often relieve positive symptoms but do not have a significant impact on negative symptoms.

   b. atypical antipsychotics relieve only negative symptoms.

   c. atypical antipsychotics tend to cause many more extrapyramidal side effects than do the typical antipsychotics.

   d. typical antipsychotics cause blood dyscrasias, whereas atypical ones do not.

8. What is the difference between assertive community treatment (ACT) and intensive case management (ICM)?

   a. ACT programs are more comprehensive than ICM programs and provide an individualized program of care delivered within the client's community by a team of professionals to clients who are identified as "high need."

   b. ICM programs use pairs of managers to intervene with clients who are at high risk for relapse.

   c. ACT programs are cheaper than ICM programs.

   d. ICM programs are more of an umbrella approach to care delivery, using community resources such as schools and churches to help provide care.

9. Assessment of violence potential is an important part of nursing care on the inpatient unit. Which of the following is *not* an indicator that Richard, a client with schizophrenia, may be at high risk for violence while in the hospital?

   a. Richard assaulted an officer prior to his admission.

b. Richard reports feeling that everyone on the unit is "out to get me."

c. Richard has never used drugs or alcohol.

d. Richard is suspicious of the nursing staff.

10. Sharon states, "I can see someone sticking out from underneath my bed, and he's telling me that I need to be killed!" Your most therapeutic initial nursing response to this statement is

a. "Sharon, I don't see or hear anything, but it sounds as though you are very frightened."

b. "Sharon, just tell the man to go away."

c. "Sharon, there is no man under your bed. Let's go to the dining room now."

d. "Sharon, you are safe here, so don't worry about that."

CHAPTER 26

The Client Who Displays Angry, Aggressive, or Violent Behavior

Although the range of aggressive behaviors, including violence, occurs in all clinical diagnostic categories, certain subgroups of psychiatric diagnoses have been linked with violent behavior, such as antisocial personality disorder, paranoid schizophrenia, schizoaffective disorder, and substance abuse. Antecedent events that have been linked with client violence on inpatient units are a coercive interaction style, arguments with other clients, and arguments with staff whose behavior in the process of caring for the client is interpreted by the client as intrusive and frustrating or indifferent.

When developing a nursing care plan for the client who is at high risk for aggressive and violent behavior, the nurse gathers information, such as a history of aggressive or violent behavior and substance abuse; factors associated with increasing anxiety levels, agitation, and inclinations toward violence; cognitive appraisals of life events and aggressive responses; inability to generate alternative solutions to problems; and inability to communicate angry feelings.

When planning therapeutic interventions, the nurse and client choose desired client outcomes based on the client's needs and ability to maintain self-control of aggressive and violent inclinations. Three major types of intervention strategies are verbal, pharmacotherapeutic, and physical (seclusion and restraint), which may be used separately or in combination as indicated by client needs and treatment setting protocols, with adherence to the principles of safety and least restrictive environment.

Discharge planning should incorporate education for the client and family or significant others based on an assessment of learning needs regarding the risks and characteristics of violent behavior, de-escalation strategies, and community support resources. In addition, pertinent nursing care plan information regarding the client should be communicated to appropriate referral agencies to ensure continuity of care, effective monitoring, and support. Evaluation requires a close examination of client and nursing efforts to determine whether the client's goals and behavior outcomes were met and to decide what additional therapeutic interventions might be more effective in reinforcing the client's efforts in exerting internal control of aggressive and violent inclinations.

LEARNING OBJECTIVES

After completing the exercises in this workbook, and studying the corresponding chapter in the textbook, the student will be able to:

- Define the broad range of responses that constitute aggressive behavior, including pertinent variables related to violence.

- Discuss significant sociodemographic, inpatient, outpatient, and other ecological factors related to people who are mentally ill and prone to violence.

- Discuss the psychological, neurobiologic, and social-environmental determinants of aggression in terms of pertinent theory and research findings.

- Discuss relevant legal issues regarding the treatment of aggressive and violent clients.

- Apply nursing care guidelines to assess, diagnose, establish goals, intervene, and evaluate outcomes for clients with aggressive and violent behavior.

KEY TERMS

Aggression: Harsh physical or verbal responses that indicate rage and a potential for destructiveness.

Anger: An emotional response to perceived frustration of desires or needs.

Hostility-related variables: Emotions, attitudes, and behaviors that occur regularly and predictably in people prone to aggression and violence.

Impulsivity: A symptom of an underlying disorder or a pervasive personality trait that causes a person to perform actions with little or no regard for the consequences.

Restraint: The use of a physical or mechanical device to involuntarily restrict the free movement of all or a portion of a person's body to control his or her physical activity.

Seclusion: The placement of a client alone in a hazard-free room that is often locked and in which others can maintain direct observation of him or her.

Temperament: Constitutional or biologically based personality dispositions that are partly inherited, evident early in life, and somewhat stable across situations and over time.

Chapter Outline

KEY TOPICS

Aggressive behavior, hostility-related variables, violence: Profiles of aggressive/violent behaviors (sociodemographic, inpatient and outpatient factors, family factors)

Determinants of aggression: Neurobiology, psychology (temperament, cognitive), social-environmental factors

Interdisciplinary goals and treatment: Verbal interventions; limit setting; cognitive interventions (guided discovery, anger management); behavioral therapy; group/family therapies; pharmacological interventions; seclusion and restraint; outpatient management

Nursing process: Assessment, diagnosis, planning, implementation (maintaining safety, defusing anger and aggression; setting limits; teaching anger management and coping skills); evaluation

■ Exercises

CASE STUDY EXERCISE

Shawn J., age 23, is admitted for psychiatric evaluation after stalking his girlfriend for 3 weeks. He was found hiding outside her door in the bushes with a knife in his hand and was brought to the emergency department by the police. Shawn is unemployed and lives with his mother. He finished the 10th grade in high school. When he was in first grade, Shawn was shy, fearful, and withdrawn whenever he was placed in a new situation. His mother states, "I think he had a seizure in third grade, but I really don't remember. It seems he was on medication for a while, but then he stopped." His mother reports that Shawn has a history of violence toward others, including herself. When he was in sixth grade, his mother found him tying up the family cat downstairs in the basement and torturing the animal. She says she had a very difficult time getting him to stop. More recently Shawn has often become involved in fist-fights at the local bar and is brought home often by his "drinking buddy" Joe. About 6 months prior to this hospitalization, he was in an automobile accident and suffered a concussion, for which he was observed for 3 days in the hospital. After clearance, he was discharged and states, "I haven't had any problems since then."

1. Using Box 24-8 in Textbook Chapter 24, list areas of assessment for Shawn's violent behavior, and discuss evidence you have gathered so far from his history.

2. Using Box 26-1 in Textbook Chapter 26, list the factors that you have already assessed from the above history that place Shawn at risk for violent behavior.

3. Explain how Shawn's history would be considered by a clinician using the temperament theory as an explanation for his violent potential.

On the unit, Shawn spends the first 2 days in his room. When he begins to venture out, he argues with clients regarding use of games and equipment, and which TV channel to watch. He is often heard raising his voice and yelling at others. During one of your shifts, you ask Shawn to go to the dining room for lunch, and he responds, "Listen, Miss Right, I'm going to tell you a thing or two: you don't push me around! I don't care who you are!"

4. What would be your most therapeutic nursing intervention in response to Shawn's outburst?

5. The psychiatrist believes that Shawn may have low serotonin syndrome. Discuss the theory of low serotonin syndrome, and include mention of the following neurotransmitters: 5HT, DA, HVA, NE, 5HIAA, MHPG, and MAO.

6. List three potential medications that could help Shawn control his aggressive outbursts. Provide the medication name, classification, dosage range for Shawn, indications for using the medication, and cautions (refer to Table 26-1 in the textbook).

Shawn is invited to the unit group, "Anger Management and Coping Skills." He reluctantly agrees to attend the group, but notes, "I've never been in a group, and I really don't think I'll do very well. Are you trying to tell me that I'm a bad person?" After talking with Shawn about the goals of the group, he states, "Oh, this sounds like a real great idea: put me in a room with six other people, and 'Let's see how Shawnie does!' I don't want to go. What am I angry about, anyway?"

7. Using cognitive theory, discuss the role that Shawn's attributions may play in his anger about attending the group.

8. Discuss goals that the group therapist will have for the anger management group.

One day, following a group session, you notice Shawn pacing the hallway with his hands clenched, muttering, "This is a bunch of crap!" He then enters the TV room and tells the two clients who are watching a show, "I'm changing it to the sports channel," which he then does. When the clients respond by complaining, Shawn erupts into an outburst, saying, "You watch TV all day, and I never get to! I'm putting it where I want, and if you don't like it, you can go to hell!" You then enter the TV room.

9. Describe cues that Shawn's aggressiveness was escalating in the above situation.

10. Where might you have intervened earlier to diffuse his anger?

11. Discuss verbal intervention strategies that you can use with Shawn at this time.

12. How would you position yourself in the TV room, and how would you ensure that you are safe while confronting Shawn?

Shawn's behavior continues to escalate. You remove the other clients from the TV room and call for help. When two additional staff arrive, Shawn picks up a chair and holds it toward the staff with the legs out. He makes shoving motions with the chair and says, "Back off, or I'll throw this damn chair straight through the window!" Shawn does not respond to verbal interventions by staff to calm him, nor will he accept medications. He refuses to take a time-out in his room but continues to yell obscenities at staff while brandishing the chair. Staff proceed to restrain Shawn.

13. Discuss the HCFA guidelines for using restraints and seclusion in inpatient settings.

14. Was restraining Shawn appropriate, given this scenario?

15. After the restraints have been removed and Shawn is placed back in the milieu, discuss ways that staff can cope with their own anxiety and feelings about what occurred.

CRITICAL THINKING AND SELF-EVALUATION EXERCISES

1. Have you been in a situation in which you felt afraid or threatened by another person? Describe your emotional feelings and your cognitive thoughts. How might you provide comfort for yourself following such an event?

2. When you read the above case scenario, what were your thoughts or feelings about what was happening?

■ NCLEX-Style Exam Questions

1. Which of the following best describes the main differences between anger and violence?
   a. Anger is a normal human emotional response to perceived frustration of desires or needs; violence is a destructive physical or verbal response to anger.
   b. Anger is an abnormally exaggerated response to aggression.
   c. Violence is adaptive if used in the appropriate place and time and as an appropriate response to aggressive behavior.
   d. Violence is never an adaptive response under any circumstance.

2. Which of the following is *not* a general criterion that characterizes impulse-control disorders?
   a. Inability to control impulses to behave in ways that are harmful toward self or others
   b. Sense of excitement, gratification, or tension relief after a violent act
   c. Sense of increasing pressure, discomfort, or energy before acting on an impulse
   d. Verbalization of what is causing the impulse to harm someone else prior to doing so

3. Which of the following staff behaviors has been found to be particularly provocative when working with clients who are predisposed to aggressive or violent behavior?
   a. Asking personal questions when they are inappropriate
   b. Engaging in disputes over medication, supplies, or rules on the unit
   c. Providing the client with a list of possible goals for behavior change
   d. Talking excessively with the client in front of other clients

4. In a study about clients who had physically attacked someone before inpatient hospitalization for violent behavior, which of the following was found to have occurred 56% of the time?
   a. Strangers were the victims of these attacks.
   b. Victims of the attacks were alcoholic.
   c. Family members were the object of these attacks.
   d. The client had used some weapon of force.

5. Neurobiologic factors are increasingly being explored as an explanation for aggressive behavior. Which of the following is true?
   a. Temperament theory is one of the leading hypotheses for violent behavior.
   b. There have been no links between neurotransmitters and aggression.
   c. Aggressive behavior is associated with clients who later contract Parkinson's disease.
   d. Brain neuroimaging studies show that aggressive behavior is linked to damage of brain structures located in the limbic, frontal, and temporal lobes.

6. You have been working on anger management with your client, Sharon. She yells during dinner, "Give me that salt shaker!" What is the best nursing intervention at this time?
   a. "Sharon, you need to stop yelling right now and ask for the salt in the correct manner."
   b. "Sharon, you may have the salt after you ask for it in the way that we talked about earlier."
   c. "Sharon, it's not appropriate for you to ask for the salt that way; besides, you are on a low-salt diet right now."
   d. "Sharon, what do you think is wrong with the way you are asking for the salt?"

7. Joseph is very manipulative and has pushed the limits since his arrival on your unit. His care plan includes a break for cigarettes every hour during the afternoon if he follows his behavioral plan to attend the morning group on anger management. He asks you, "I couldn't get to my

group this morning because I overslept. Can I just this one time go for a cigarette now?" What is the most therapeutic nursing intervention?

a. "Well, I know you were tired from last night. You can go at 2 p.m."

b. "No, Joe. Your plan says that you need to attend that group in order to have cigarette breaks."

c. "Why do you think you should be allowed to go for a break?"

d. "Joe, let's review your care plan and discuss whether or not it needs to be revised."

8. You are leading an anger management group in your inpatient program. Mark says during the group, "I'm feeling really tense, and I'm fidgety today." What is your best response to Mark?

a. "Mark, can you talk more about those feelings, and what they are like?"

b. "Mark, why don't you and I just do a very quick relaxation intervention to calm you down before we go on with group today?"

c. "Could it be that it's because we started late, and Susan was late again, which you pointed out yesterday makes you angry?"

d. "Susan, how do you feel about Mark's statement?"

9. Written orders for restraint or seclusion for psychiatric–mental health clients are limited to

a. 4 hours for adults; 2 hours for children and adolescents aged 9 to 17; 1 hour for children under 9 years old.

b. 6 hours for adults and adolescents; 2 hours for children; 1 hour for children under 9.

c. 12 hours for adults; 6 for children and adolescents aged 9 to 17; 4 hours for children under 9.

d. 24 hours for adults; 12 for children and adolescents.

10. When the client is in restraint or seclusion, which of the following must occur?

a. He or she must be given water at least every 2 hours.

b. He or she must be fed at least every 2 hours.

c. He or she must be monitored continually.

d. He or she must be seen by a physician or licensed independent practitioner within the first 3 hours of initiation of seclusion or restraint.

CHAPTER 27

The Client Who Abuses Drugs and Alcohol

Substance use disorders include both substance abuse and substance dependency. *Substance abuse* occurs when an individual uses alcohol or other drugs repeatedly to the extent that functional problems occur. *Substance dependency* is diagnosed when the individual continues using alcohol or other drugs in spite of negative consequences, such as significant functional problems in daily living.

The substance abuse disorders are classified by 12 categories of substances: alcohol, amphetamines, caffeine, cannabis, cocaine, hallucinogens, inhalants, nicotine, opioids, phencyclidine, sedative-hypnotics, and polysubstance abuse. All of the substance abuse disorders may be associated with any of the common subdiagnoses of dependence (abuse, intoxication, and withdrawal). Substance abuse disorders are multidimensional and related strongly to neurophysiological processes as well as to psychosocial and behavioral processes.

Alcohol abuse and alcohol dependency are among the most serious public health problems in the United States. The incidence and consequences of alcohol-related accidents resulting in fatalities or permanent injuries are enormous. Many American children and adolescents suffer from the effects of drug and alcohol abuse in multiple areas of functioning, and the incidence and prevalence of substance abuse disorders are high in adolescents. Many clients suffer from dual diagnosis (coexistence of a substance abuse disorder and a major psychiatric disorder).

Interdisciplinary treatment of the client with a substance abuse disorder is critical to a successful recovery process and includes detoxification programs and facilities, inpatient rehabilitation, outpatient programs, and private practice physician treatment. In addition, there is a wide network of 12-step treatment programs throughout the world.

The nurse plays a critical role in the treatment and management of the client with substance abuse or withdrawal from substances. The major issues in care of the client who is admitted for substance abuse include maintaining the client's safety; breaking through denial; managing anxiety; teaching effective coping strategies; improving family processes; enhancing self-esteem; and promoting healthy activities. Frequent re-evaluation and assessment, with appropriate changes in care, are necessary to enhance treatment and to ensure that clients move toward healthier lifestyles that are free of substances of abuse.

LEARNING OBJECTIVES

After completing the exercises in this workbook, and studying the corresponding chapter in the textbook, the student will be able to:

- Define "substance abuse" and "dependency."

- Explain current diagnostic categorization of various types of substance abuse and dependency disorders.

- Discuss the common etiological concepts related to substance abuse and dependency.

- Discuss the incidence and significance of substance abuse and dependency.

- Discuss the importance of recognizing dual diagnoses and comorbidity in clients with substance abuse and dependency, and the implications for prognosis.

- Describe the effects of substance abuse disorders on physiology, behavior, society, and the family.

- Discuss interdisciplinary treatment interventions for the client with a substance abuse disorder.

- Apply the components of the nursing process to the client who abuses or is dependent on substances.

KEY TERMS

Alcohol (ethanol): A legal chemical substance (drug) that commonly leads to abuse and dependency.

Blackout: A phenomenon in which a person functions normally while drinking but later has no memory of what occurred during that period, with no accompanying loss of consciousness.

Blood alcohol level (BAL): Milligrams of alcohol per milliliter of blood.

Club drugs: A group of synthetic drugs used commonly in nightclubs and as recreational drugs.

Delirium tremens (DTs): Most serious form of withdrawal from alcohol; occurs after cessation or reduction in prolonged heavy drinking; can be a medical emergency and needs immediate treatment.

Dual diagnosis: A diagnosis of a coexisting substance abuse or dependency disorder and a major psychiatric disorder; the disorders are unrelated and meet the *DSM-IV-TR* diagnostic criteria for each specific disorder.

Fetal alcohol syndrome: A syndrome characterized by a group of congenital birth defects caused by the mother's drinking while pregnant.

Proof: Concentration of ethyl alcohol in a beverage.

Substance abuse: Use of alcohol or other drugs repeatedly to the extent that functional problems occur; does not include compulsive use or addiction.

Substance dependency: Continued used of alcohol or other drugs despite negative consequences, such as significant functional problems in daily living.

Tolerance: A phenomenon that occurs after heavy drug or alcohol use in which the user needs more of the drug to achieve the same effect.

Wernicke-Korsakoff syndrome: Alcoholic amnesia related to thiamine deficiency.

Chapter Outline

SUBSTANCE ABUSE AND DEPENDENCY
Historical Context
Epidemiology
Prenatal Alcohol and Drug Abuse
Cultural Considerations
Etiology
Psychosocial and Behavioral Factors
Biological Factors
Theoretical Concepts
Comorbidities and Dual Diagnoses
Implications and Prognosis
Signs and Symptoms/Diagnostic Criteria
Alcohol Abuse and Dependency
   Chemical Properties of Alcohol
   Alcohol Concentration in the Body
   Tolerance
   Blackout

Alcohol-Induced Disorders
   Intoxication
   Alcohol Withdrawal
   Alcoholic Hallucinosis
   Alcoholic Amnestic Disorder
   Alcoholic Dementia
Medical Consequences of Alcohol Abuse and Dependency
Controlled Substances
Interdisciplinary Treatment
Medical Detoxification from Alcohol
The Rehabilitation Process
Medications Used to Treat Drug Dependency
Self-Help Groups
APPLICATION OF THE NURSING PROCESS TO THE CLIENT WITH A SUBSTANCE-RELATED DISORDER
Assessment
Physical Examination
Psychosocial Assessment
Nursing Diagnoses
Planning
Implementation
Maintaining Safety
Breaking Through Denial
Managing Anxiety
Teaching Effective Coping Strategies
Improving Family Processes
Enhancing Self-Esteem
Promoting Healthy Activities
Evaluation

KEY TOPICS

Substance abuse and dependency: Historical context, epidemiology, prenatal alcohol and drug abuse, cultural considerations, etiology (psychosocial and behavioral factors, biological factors, theoretical concepts)

Signs and symptoms/diagnostic criteria: Alcohol abuse and dependency, chemical properties of alcohol, alcohol concentration in the body, tolerance, blackout, alcohol-induced disorders (intoxication, alcohol withdrawal, alcoholic hallucinosis, alcoholic amnestic disorder, alcoholic dementia)

Medical consequences: Alcohol abuse and dependency, controlled substances

Interdisciplinary treatment: Medical detoxification from alcohol, rehabilitation process, medications used to treat drug dependency, self-help groups

Nursing process: Assessment (physical examination, psychosocial assessment), nursing diagnoses, planning, implementation (maintaining safety, breaking through denial, managing anxiety, teaching effective coping strategies, improving family processes, enhancing self-esteem, promoting healthy activities); evaluation

■ Exercises

CASE STUDY EXERCISE

Patricia, age 29, was admitted after her husband, Jerry, found her unconscious at home. On interview, you discover that Patricia is not employed outside the home, but stays home with the couple's 5-year-old girl, Cassie, who is scheduled to begin kindergarten in 3 months. Patricia has used alcohol for over 10 years, in increasingly larger amounts. Currently, she drinks about four six-packs of beer a day while she is home during the day. About a month ago, she was offered a joint of marijuana by a neighbor; she is now smoking about four joints per day. Jerry states that during the past 2 months, Patricia has been having "blackouts," when she does not remember the events of the previous evening.

1. Discuss how you would assess Patricia's current level of alcohol and drug use. What types of tools might you be able to use?

2. List the symptoms that Patricia is having in the above scenario.

3. What is Patricia's probable *DSM-IV-TR* diagnosis? Does Patricia have a dual diagnosis, using just the information given above? Why or why not?

On the first day of her admission, Patricia begins to complain to you that she is feeling "nauseous, and my hands are shaky." You take her vital signs and find her BP to be 140/90; her pulse is 80.

4. What do you think is happening?

5. List the nursing priority for Patricia for the next week. Use the Nursing Process Worksheet on the next page to design a plan of care for addressing this priority.

6. Using Box 27-6 in Textbook Chapter 27, list three goals to be accomplished to get Patricia through the next week.

7. Describe appropriate medications that will be useful to help Patricia through the next week. Describe their classification, mechanisms of action, target symptoms, and dosage ranges.

Include nursing care for any potential side effects.

During Patricia's second week of hospitalization, she has progressed successfully through detoxification and is medically stabilized. When you talk with her about her alcoholism and drug use, Patricia states, "Well, yeah, I had a little bump in the road, but in general, I'm really fine and I don't need any more treatment. I mean, I'm a pretty independent person and can take care of myself and my family." You discuss referring Patricia to a follow-up program for alcohol and substance abuse, and she states, "I'm really too busy to do that. I have to take care of my baby, you know."

8. Discuss some strategies you might use to work with Patricia's denial.

9. In regard to Patricia's substance abuse, what is a realistic goal for her for a 2-week inpatient stay?

10. Using Textbook Table 27-3, discuss some interventions that would be used in an intensive treatment program to help Patricia to maintain sobriety and begin to address her drug use.

CRITICAL THINKING AND SELF-EVALUATION EXERCISE

1. Substance abuse is common on college campuses. Explore what your campus has to offer for students who may be having difficulty managing alcohol and drug use while in college. List the resources here.

■ NCLEX-Style Exam Questions

1. "Substance abuse" is a term that is used when
   a. a person uses drugs continuously despite negative consequences; the person does experience tolerance.
   b. a person uses any form of drug or alcohol.
   c. a person uses alcohol or drugs repeatedly, but not compulsively or addictively; the person who is abusing substances will not experience withdrawal.
   d. a person is addicted to drugs or alcohol and cannot stop using them.

NURSING PROCESS WORKSHEET

Health Problem (Title)

Related to

↓

Etiology (Related Factors)

Evidenced by

↓

**Signs and Symptoms
(Defining Characteristics)**

Client Goal*

Nursing Interventions**

Evaluative Statement

*More than one client goal may be appropriate. For this exercise, choose one client goal that demonstrates a direct resolution of the client problem identified in the nursing diagnosis.
**Be sure you are able to list the scientific rationale for each nursing intervention you order.

2. The major difference between substance abuse and substance dependency is that

   a. a person who is abusing does not have withdrawal symptoms, whereas the dependent person uses the substance despite significant functional difficulties and will have withdrawal.

   b. in substance dependence, the individual has shared with his or her significant others that there is definitely a problem.

   c. people who abuse substances are often seen by their peers as "alcoholic."

   d. people who are dependent often lose their jobs or drop out of school.

3. Which of the following is considered a "gateway" drug?

   a. Cocaine

   b. Wine

   c. Marijuana

   d. All alcohols

4. Sandra was diagnosed with cocaine abuse at age 30. When she was 23, Sandra was diagnosed with major depressive episode, and she has continued to have depression off and on since then. Which of the following is the most correct statement?

   a. Sandra is probably using cocaine in combination with her antidepressants to try to get higher.

   b. Sandra is probably using cocaine to cope with her depressive symptoms, and she would be considered to have a dual diagnosis.

   c. Sandra will need to have the cocaine abuse treated before anything can be done about her depression.

   d. Sandra will have a very poor prognosis for recovery if she discontinues cocaine, because it will enhance her depressive symptoms.

5. The rate of absorption of alcohol into the blood is affected by all except which of the following factors?

   a. Substances in the beverage

   b. The amount of physical activity the individual had prior to the drinking episode

   c. Food in the stomach

   d. The drinker's emotional state

6. John began drinking a six-pack of beer every day in his freshman year of college. By his sophomore year, he is drinking two six-packs to get the same effect. This phenomenon is best described as

   a. alcohol abuse.

   b. intoxication.

   c. tolerance.

   d. dependence.

7. Shaundra was admitted to the emergency department for intoxication with alcohol. She has an unsteady gait, myopathy, and neuropathy, and cannot remember past or recent events. When treated with thiamine, her symptoms greatly improve. Shaundra is most likely suffering from

   a. scurvy.

   b. alcohol dependence with memory impairment.

   c. Wernicke Korsakoff syndrome.

   d. alcoholic dementia.

8. George is admitted to the detoxification unit on Sunday evening. His withdrawal symptoms from alcohol are most likely to begin, and he will likely need the most support, at what time?

   a. Monday morning

   b. Tuesday evening

   c. Wednesday morning

   d. Friday evening

9. The recommended first-line pharmacological agents for managing severe alcohol withdrawal symptoms are

   a. serotonin reuptake inhibitors.

   b. atypical antipsychotics.

   c. benzodiazepines.

   d. major tranquilizers.

10. Safety is the nursing priority for a client who is at risk for alcohol withdrawal. A care plan for the client who is in withdrawal must include

   a. observation for symptoms; vital signs; seizure and fall precautions; medications as ordered.

   b. vital signs; medications as prescribed.

   c. suicide precautions, because suicide attempts are frequent during withdrawal.

   d. seizure precautions and vital signs.

CHAPTER 28

The Client With a Cognitive Disorder

Cognitive disorders appear not only in the aging population but also in the general population. The possible etiologies of cognitive disorders include primary brain disease, systemic disturbances, influences of exogenous substances, and withdrawal and residual effects of exogenous substances. Aberrant behaviors associated with these disorders may include deficits in the sensorium, attention span, orientation, perception, and memory. Symptoms of cognitive disorders may be approached in terms of acute onset and chronic progression. Gathering and analyzing assessment data for a client with a cognitive disorder requires the participation of family members or friends who have been in close contact with the client.

Continuity of care involves the collaborative efforts of the entire interdisciplinary healthcare team. Goal setting for the client with an organic disorder focuses on eliminating the organic etiology, preventing acceleration of symptoms, and preserving dignity. Specific nursing interventions strive to maintain the client's optimal physical health, structure the environment, promote socialization and independent functioning, and preserve the family unit.

LEARNING OBJECTIVES

After completing the exercises in this workbook, and studying the corresponding chapter in the textbook, the student will be able to:

- Define the term "cognitive mental disorder."

- Discuss the incidence and significance of cognitive disorders.

- Identify the clinical features or behaviors associated with various cognitive disorders.

- Compare the possible etiologies of the various cognitive disorders.

- Explain the continuum of care and interdisciplinary treatments for clients and family members affected by the assorted cognitive disorders.

- Discuss the treatment interventions typically initiated for clients with various cognitive disorders.

- Apply the steps of the nursing process to clients with any of the cognitive disorders.

KEY TERMS

Agnosia: Inability to recognize or identify familiar objects (eg, the parts of a telephone).

Aphasia: Difficulty finding the appropriate words in conversation.

Apraxia: Inability to perform motor tasks despite intact motor function.

Cognitive mental disorders: Group of disorders characterized by a disruption of or deficit in cognitive functioning.

Confabulation: A characteristic of cognitive disorders in which an affected individual fills in gaps in memory with fabricated or imagined data.

Delirium: A cognitive disorder caused by an acute disruption of brain homeostasis that is characterized by a rapid onset of cognitive dysfunction and disruption in consciousness; when the cause of that disruption is eliminated or subsides, the cognitive deficits usually resolve within a few days or sometimes weeks.

Dementia: A cognitive disorder resulting from primary brain pathology that is usually not amenable to treatment; prognosis depends on whether the cause can be identified and the condition reversed.

Sundowning: A characteristic feature of dementia in which most behavior changes are more pronounced in the evenings, after sunset.

Chapter Outline

DELIRIUM
Etiology
Signs and Symptoms/Diagnostic Criteria
Implications and Prognosis

KEY TOPICS

Delirium

Nursing process in delirium: Assessment, diagnosis, planning, implementation (managing confusion; providing safety; helping with personal care; providing client and family education); Evaluation

Types of dementia: Alzheimer's disease; vascular dementia; Parkinson's disease; Huntington's chorea; HIV; Pick's disease; Creutzfeldt-Jakob disease

Nursing process in dementia: Assessment, diagnosis, planning, implementation (managing health; enhancing sensory capabilities; meeting physical needs; encouraging appropriate behaviors; preventing injury; preserving families)

Amnestic disorders

■ Exercises

CASE STUDY EXERCISE

Harvey T., age 55, is admitted to your unit for psychiatric evaluation. Harvey has been a bank courier for 35 years, a stable, dependent employee who is well liked by all his coworkers. His wife describes Harvey as a handsome, clean-cut, attractive man who has always paid attention to his appearance. Harvey was admitted following an episode in which he called his wife, Mildred, on his cellular phone to ask for directions back to their city. He had left for work that morning and ended up in a city 50 miles from their home. On the phone, he was tearful and anxious, and had had a minor fender-bender. Mildred and Harvey have been married for 30 years and have enjoyed a good quality of life.

Mildred is very anxious about Harvey's admission, fearful that perhaps he has a brain tumor. She is present during the intake assessment and relates that in the past year, she has noticed that Harvey has begun to have trouble remembering his work schedule. Just recently, over the past 2 to 3 months, he has begun to appear disheveled and unkempt; sometimes "he doesn't even shave before he leaves for work! I have to remind him." He has been calling her from the cellular phone for directions to work for about a week. Mildred says, "He never was very good with directions, so I didn't really think anything about it at first." She also says that recently Harvey has become more short-tempered, particularly at work, and on several occasions has shouted at and argued with his supervisor.

1. Using Box 28-4 in Textbook Chapter 28, list the elements you will include in a comprehensive assessment of Harvey's functional status. Include the data you have gathered thus far.

2. Describe at least one formal assessment tool that you can use to assess Harvey's cognitive status on admission.

During the interview, you observe that Harvey appears uninterested at times. When he is asked why he was admitted, he does not answer and shrugs his shoulders. He mentions that he is "sad" about being here, engaging in the conversation for only very brief periods at a time. While you are interviewing Harvey, you actually begin to feel sad yourself.

3. Using the Nursing Process Worksheet on the following page, design a plan for caring for Harvey during the first 24 hours of his admission. What would be your primary nursing goal.

4. What data do you have from the above clinical scenario that Harvey may be aphasic?

On the second day of Harvey's stay, you assess that he cannot dress himself; he comes out for breakfast with his shorts placed backward. When you observe him in the bathroom, you note that he cannot shave or brush his teeth. He picks up the toothbrush and stands looking in the mirror. In the dining room, one of the clients asked Harvey to pass the salt and pepper, and Harvey passed a napkin.

5. Describe an example of apraxia that Harvey displayed.

6. Describe an example of agnosia that Harvey displayed.

7. Describe an example of decreased executive functioning that Harvey displayed.

8. List *DSM-IV-TR* symptoms that confirm to you that Harvey is suffering from dementia of the Alzheimer's type.

9. Discuss medications that may be helpful to Harvey. Include the classification, mechanism of action, dosage, side effects, and teaching points.

Harvey has been on the unit for 3 weeks, and the additional structure, medications, and support have increased his ability to perform his activities of daily living. His confusion has decreased somewhat. His wife is sad about his diagnosis of Alzheimer's but is encouraged by his progress. She is very happy that she will be able to take Harvey back home. You prepare the couple for discharge.

10. Using Table 28-2 in Textbook Chapter 28, describe the symptoms that provide evidence of what stage Alzheimer's disease Harvey has.

11. What will you do in regard to patient education prior to the couple's departure?

12. Discuss the potential for "caregiver burnout" for Mildred. How might you help her to gain support once Harvey has left the hospital?

CRITICAL THINKING AND SELF-EVALUATION EXERCISE

Do a search on the Internet for "Alzheimer's disease" and see what you find. Do you believe it would be difficult for a lay caregiver such as Mildred (Harvey's wife in the above clinical scenario) to access helpful information about this disease? What are the barriers to lay caregivers in getting assistance and support in caring for their loved ones?

■ NCLEX-Style Exam Questions

1. Jean has early Alzheimer's disease. When asked about her family history, she relates that she has two children who are both grown and who visit her around the holidays each year. You subsequently discover that Jean has one child who is currently assigned overseas and has not been home for 2 years. Which of the following would best describe Jean's behavior?

   a. Jean is confabulating, most likely to cover for her memory deficit.
   b. Jean is confused about her children and needs refocusing.
   c. Jean demonstrates aphasia when discussing her children.
   d. Jean is showing signs of agnosia in that she is unable to name her children.

2. Delirium is different from many other cognitive disorders in that
   a. it has a slow onset, but if caught early it can be treated with medications.

NURSING PROCESS WORKSHEET

Health Problem (Title)

Client Goal*

Related to
↓

Etiology (Related Factors)

Nursing Interventions**

Evidenced by
↓

**Signs and Symptoms
(Defining Characteristics)**

Evaluative Statement

*More than one client goal may be appropriate. For this exercise, choose one client goal that demonstrates a direct resolution of the client problem identified in the nursing diagnosis.
**Be sure you are able to list the scientific rationale for each nursing intervention you order.

b. it is much less responsive to pharmacological treatment than the other disorders.

c. it has a rapid onset and is highly treatable if diagnosed quickly.

d. it is characterized by a period of disorganization and confusion.

3. Which of the following nursing diagnoses would be most critical (ie, highest priority) for the client experiencing acute delirium?

a. Acute confusion related to delirium of known/unknown etiology

b. Risk for injury related to confusion and cognitive deficits

c. Fall precautions related to acute confusion

d. Risk for self-mutilation related to confusion and cognitive deficits

4. Parkinson's disease is thought to be caused by

a. a deficit in the postsynaptic receptors for dopamine, resulting in a deficit of that neurotransmitter in the synapse.

b. overproduction of dopa, which responds to treatment with its antagonist, L-dopa.

c. a decreased number of brain cells in the substantia nigra, resulting in dopamine depletion.

d. too many dopamine receptors in the cerebellum.

5. Major goals for the nursing care of clients with dementia include that the client will

a. be safe and eat appropriately.

b. be safe; be physiologically stable; have infrequent episodes of agitation.

c. be physically stable; maintain normal body weight; be safe.

d. have no self-harm behaviors; maintain sleep and appetite.

6. Susan has advanced Alzheimer's disease and becomes confused at mealtimes. She has agnosia, apraxia, and disturbed executive functioning. Which of the following is the most appropriate nursing intervention?

a. Provide Susan with her tray, opening containers for her.

b. Ask Susan what she would like from the buffet, and give her finger foods.

c. Provide Susan with her tray, but encourage her to open her own packages.

d. Have Susan eat in her room to avoid distractions while eating.

7. Tacrine (Cognex) is a drug that is used in clients with cognitive disorders. Tacrine works mainly by

a. increasing levels of dopamine in the substantia nigra.

b. elevating levels of acetylcholine (ACH) in the system by decreasing binding sites of acetylcholinesterase.

c. reducing levels of acetylcholine in the system.

d. elevating alanine aminotransferase (ALT) levels in the liver.

8. When giving tacrine (Cognex) to an elderly client, the nurse must be aware that

a. since the liver is most vulnerable to tacrine, liver function tests must be done periodically.

b. the client will suffer from dry mouth and difficulty urinating.

c. the most common side effects are headache and dizziness, so the client must be monitored for falls.

d. tacrine works only in clients with late-stage dementia.

9. The hallmark of amnestic disorders is

a. long-term memory is affected most.

b. this class of disorders does not involve memory loss.

c. clients with these disorders tend to confabulate.

d. short-term memory loss.

10. A 65-year-old man has been admitted to the ICU following surgical resection of the bowel. He has developed a fever. In addition to treating the fever, nurses also monitor the man for signs of delirium. Which of the following behaviors might indicate that he is becoming delirious?

a. He cannot brush his teeth.

b. He removes his surgical bandage and begins picking at his sheets.

c. He identifies his fork as a spoon.

d. He has trouble remembering his birth date.

CHAPTER 29

Working With Pediatric Clients

The effects of child and adolescent mental illness include both direct and indirect costs: the increased likelihood of the disorder continuing into later life, feelings of guilt and blame, unmet needs of siblings and other family members, marital stress and conflict, and diminished productivity of lives. Factors placing the child or adolescent at risk for the development of mental health disorders include biological factors (eg, family history of a mental illness, immature development of the brain, and brain abnormality); psychological factors (eg, family problems and dysfunction); and stressors (eg, poverty, mentally ill or substance-abusing parents, teen parents, abuse, discrimination due to race, creed, or color, chronic parental conflict or divorced parents, and chronic illness or disability).

Children and adolescents are affected by many psychiatric illnesses, including those that are usually first diagnosed during infancy, childhood, or adolescence and those that, although common in adults, have different manifestations and require different treatment in children and adolescents. The most common psychiatric illnesses of the pediatric population are ADHD, conduct disorder, ODD, adjustment disorder, OCD, phobias, social anxiety disorder, generalized anxiety disorder, separation anxiety disorder, PTSD, depression, bipolar disorder, autism-spectrum disorders, eating disorders, substance abuse, trichotillomania, and tic disorders.

Early intervention with children and adolescents at risk can prevent more serious mental disturbance later in life. Child and adolescent mental illness is treated by biological interventions, such as psychotropic medication, and by psychosocial interventions, such as therapies, therapeutic approaches designed for each client, school modifications, and community-based services. The role of the nurse in child and adolescent mental health care is essential. The nurse performs a thorough assessment, including assessment of family functioning, current problems, history, and a mental status examination. The nurse also provides medication education, meets the needs of the families, and promotes the rights of children in treatment settings, which includes avoiding seclusion and restraints and providing advocacy.

Nursing care of the child with ADHD focuses on the family as a whole and involves educating the child and family about treatment and behavioral strategies, helping the family cope, managing developmental and academic issues, teaching social skills, and improving self-esteem.

LEARNING OBJECTIVES

After completing the exercises in this workbook, and studying the corresponding chapter in the textbook, the student will be able to:

- Discuss the effects of childhood mental illness.

- Identify factors that contribute to psychiatric disorders in children and adolescents.

- Describe general interventions available for children or adolescents with psychiatric disorders.

- Discuss the role of the psychiatric–mental health nurse in child and adolescent mental health care.

- Apply the nursing process to the care of children and adolescents with ADHD.

- Identify the most common childhood psychiatric illnesses.

- Discuss psychiatric nursing care for the child or adolescent facing a serious medical illness.

KEY TERMS

Adjustment disorder: A psychiatric disorder marked by clinically or behaviorally significant symptoms that develop within 3 months after the onset of an identifiable stressor.

Advocacy: Formal or informal promotion of children's rights.

Anhedonia: Loss of pleasure in hobbies or activities of interest; a characteristic of depression.

Attention-deficit disorder (ADD): A psychiatric disorder characterized by inattention without hyperactivity or impulsivity.

Attention-deficit hyperactivity disorder (ADHD): A psychiatric disorder characterized by inattention, impulsiveness, and hyperactivity.

Autism: A genetic disorder of neuronal organization that requires early detection and treatment.

Double depression: A diagnosis given when dysthymia and major depression occur together.

Dysthymia: A mild form of depression that lasts 1 year or more in a child or adolescent.

Obsessive–compulsive disorder: A disorder characterized by recurrent intrusive thoughts (obsessions) and repetitive behaviors (compulsions) that the client realizes are senseless but feels he or she must perform.

Oppositional-defiant disorder (ODD): A psychiatric disorder marked by negativistic, defiant behaviors such as stubbornness, resistance to directions, and unwillingness to negotiate with adults or peers.

Phobias: Morbid, irrational, and persistent fears.

Separation anxiety disorder: A childhood psychiatric disorder in which a child experiences severe anxiety to the point of panic when separated from a parent or attachment figure.

Systems of care: A comprehensive spectrum of mental health and other necessary services organized into a coordinated network.

Tic: A sudden repetitive movement, gesture, or utterance.

Tourette syndrome: The most severe tic disorder, characterized by multiple motor tics and one or more vocal tics many times throughout the day for 1 year or more.

Trichotillomania: A chronic impulse-control condition in which clients have an irresistible urge to pull out their hair; they feel tension before pulling out the hair and relief or pleasure during and after pulling.

Chapter Outline

OVERVIEW OF MENTAL HEALTH AND PSYCHIATRIC DISORDERS IN CHILDREN AND ADOLESCENTS
Theories of Child Development
Psychoanalytic Perspectives
   Sigmund Freud's Psychosexual Theory
   Erik Erikson's Psychosocial Theory
Piaget's Cognitive-Developmental Theory
Contemporary Approaches to Child Development
Risk Factors for Child and Adolescent Mental Disorders
Biological Influences
Psychosocial Influences
Stressors
   Divorce
   Child Abuse
Protective/Resilient Influences for Mental Health in Children and Adolescents
General Interventions for Child and Adolescent Mental Disorders

The Interdisciplinary Team and Coordination of Care
   Treatment Settings and Continuum of Care
   Wrap-Around Services and Systems of Care
     Approaches
Prevention and Early Identification
Types of Therapies
Special Education
Community-Based Services
Pharmacological Therapy
Nursing Care
   Assessment
     Family Functioning
     Current Problem
     History
     Mental Status Examination
   Interventions
     Providing Medication Education
     Meeting Families' Needs
     Promoting the Rights of Children in Treatment Settings
     Avoiding Seclusion and Restraint
     Providing Advocacy
ATTENTION-DEFICIT HYPERACTIVITY DISORDER/ATTENTION-DEFICIT DISORDER
Etiology
Signs and Symptoms/Diagnostic Criteria
Comorbidities
Interdisciplinary Goals and Treatment
Pharmacological Therapy
Psychosocial Interventions
APPLICATION OF THE NURSING PROCESS TO A CLIENT WITH ADHD
Assessment
Nursing Diagnosis
Planning
Implementation
Educating the Family about Treatment and Behavioral Strategies
Helping Families Cope
Managing Developmental and Academic Issues
Teaching Social Skills
Improving Self-Esteem
Evaluation
OPPOSITIONAL-DEFIANT DISORDER
CONDUCT DISORDER
ADJUSTMENT DISORDERS
ANXIETY DISORDERS
OBSESSIVE–COMPULSIVE DISORDER
PHOBIAS
SOCIAL ANXIETY DISORDER (SOCIAL PHOBIA)
GENERALIZED ANXIETY DISORDER
SEPARATION ANXIETY DISORDER
POST-TRAUMATIC STRESS DISORDER
MOOD DISORDERS
DEPRESSION
Etiology
Signs and Symptoms
Comorbidities
Prevention

Interdisciplinary Goals and Treatment
Cognitive-Behavioral and Family Therapy
Pharmacological Therapy
BIPOLAR DISORDER
Etiology
Signs and Symptoms
Interdisciplinary Goals and Treatment
Importance of Early Identification and Treatment
Pharmacological Therapy
AUTISM-SPECTRUM DISORDERS
AUTISM
ASPERGER SYNDROME
Interdisciplinary Goals and Treatment
EATING DISORDERS
SUBSTANCE ABUSE
Etiology
Prevention of Drug and Alcohol Abuse
Interdisciplinary Goals and Treatment
TIC DISORDERS
TRICHOTILLOMANIA
SUICIDE
Signs
Prevention
Interdisciplinary Goals and Treatment
CHILDREN WITH MEDICAL ILLNESS OR DISABILITY
APPLICATION OF THE NURSING PROCESS TO THE
   CHILD OR ADOLESCENT WITH MEDICAL ILLNESS OR
   DISABILITY
Assessment
Characteristics of the Disease
Family Assessment
Nursing Diagnosis
Planning
Implementation
Evaluation
NURSES' SELF-CARE

KEY TOPICS

Theories of child development: Psychoanalytic (Freud, Erikson); Piaget; contemporary approaches

Risk factors for child and adolescent mental disorders: Biological, psychosocial, stress

Interventions for child and adolescent mental disorders: Coordinating care (treatment settings, continuums, and systems; wrap-around care); prevention and early diagnosis; therapy types; special education; community-based services; pharmacological therapy

Nursing care: Assessment, interventions (medication, family needs, children's rights, avoiding seclusion and restraint; providing advocacy)

Common psychiatric disorders: Disruptive behavior disorders; attention-deficit hyperactivity disorder and attention-deficit disorder; oppositional-defiant disorder; conduct disorder; adjustment disorders; anxiety disorders; mood disorders (depression, bipolar);

autism-spectrum disorders, eating disorders, substance abuse, tic disorders, trichotillomania, suicide, medical illness or disability

Nursing process: Assessment (characteristics of the disease, family assessment); diagnosis, planning, implementation, evaluation

Nurses' self-care

■ Exercises

CASE STUDY EXERCISE

Jana, age 11, is in sixth grade and lives at home with her parents and two siblings (5-year-old brother Jake, 6-month-old sister Kara). Jana has been admitted to the inpatient child and adolescent mental health unit for a 3-day assessment. Jana's mother states that since Kara's birth, Jana has been becoming increasingly "moody and irritable. She's not doing her chores around the house, she has been waking up at night, and complaining of stomachaches. She doesn't seem to have any fun anymore, and when we go on picnics or outings, she usually just will sit and not do anything." Jana's parents are extremely worried about her recent behavior. In school last week, Jana's teacher reported to the school nurse that she was "hitting a doll, saying, 'You're a very bad little girl, and why are you angry!' In addition, the teacher reported that she saw Jana using scissors to cut the doll's arms. After talking with Jana's teacher, the school nurse called Jana's parents to ask them to come in for a conference. At that time, the teacher, nurse, and parents all agreed that Jana's behavior has been very uncharacteristic of her normal behavior, she seems very depressed, and perhaps she would benefit from having an assessment.

1. List the symptoms that Jana is displaying that indicate she may be depressed.

2. What data above would indicate that Jana is anhedonic?

3. List recent life events that you think may be contributing to Jana's current difficulty.

When she is admitted, Jana is at first shy and withdrawn on the unit. She is observed to be avoiding meals and is often awake during the night crying. When she is approached by nursing staff, she responds to comforting. She is able to say that she feels sad but cannot talk further about it.

4. What are your immediate priorities for Jana's nursing care on admission?

5. Using the Nursing Process Worksheet on the next page, plan Jana's care for her first 24 hours on the unit.

After 2 days on the unit, Jana has begun to brighten and play with the other children. She is eating, and sleeping during the night. She states that she misses her baby sister and her brother. Her parents have been very involved in Jana's care and have come daily for parent meetings. They are interested in continued treatment for Jana following discharge.

6. Discuss at least two treatment approaches that might be useful for ongoing therapy for Jana and her family.

7. Do you believe Jana needs psychotropic medications? Why or why not?

8. Discuss Jana's developmental stage according to Erikson and Piaget, and talk about what effect an unresolved depression might have on Jana's further development.

9. What do you believe are the most important needs Jana's parents have prior to Jana's discharge?

CRITICAL THINKING AND SELF-EVALUATION EXERCISES

1. Consider for a moment the notion of a depressed child. Answer the question, "What does a child have to be depressed about?"

2. Do you believe childhood mental health disorders are spoken about and addressed adequately in American culture? In your own culture? Why or why not?

■ NCLEX-Style Exam Questions

1. In regard to the rate of recovery from a single episode of major depression in children and adolescents, which of the following is true?

a. Seventy to eighty percent of youth with depression can be treated effectively, and the recovery rate is relatively high.

b. Children and adolescents do not respond as well as adults to interventions for depression.

c. The same interventions that work in adult depression are effective in childhood depression.

d. Children and adolescent depression is more superficial, and thus they recover more quickly.

2. A 7-year-old boy being treated for depression will most likely be given which of the following first-line pharmacological choice in childhood depression?

a. Benzodiazepines

b. Tricyclic antidepressants

c. Monoamine oxidase inhibitors

d. Serotonin reuptake inhibitors

3. A 22-year-old woman states, "I just don't know who I am." Which stage of development, according to Erikson, would she have had difficulty completing?

a. Autonomy vs. shame and doubt

b. Basic trust vs. mistrust

c. Industry vs. inferiority

d. Identity vs. identity diffusion

4. It is evident that Jim has entered Piaget's stage of formal operations when he

a. speaks about a recent ballad as being reflective of his life story.

b. expresses sadness about the loss of his dog.

c. can sleep through the night without having enuresis.

d. talks about humans being homo sapiens.

5. Sandy, age 4 years, is going to the pediatrician for an injection. She asks her mother if the doctor is going to cut her arm off with the needle. Sandy is expressing the following common fear characteristic of the preschool age:

a. fear of pain.

b. fear of the unknown.

c. fear of body mutilation.

d. fear of body injury.

NURSING PROCESS WORKSHEET

Health Problem (Title)	Client Goal*

Related to

↓

Etiology (Related Factors)	Nursing Interventions**

Evidenced by

↓

Signs and Symptoms (Defining Characteristics)	Evaluative Statement

*More than one client goal may be appropriate. For this exercise, choose one client goal that demonstrates a direct resolution of the client problem identified in the nursing diagnosis.
**Be sure you are able to list the scientific rationale for each nursing intervention you order.

6. Preschool programs that target children's social and emotional competencies are an example of
   a. primary prevention.
   b. secondary prevention.
   c. tertiary prevention.
   d. quaternary prevention.

7. Kelly is being observed for ADHD. Which of the following would demonstrate that she suffers from that disorder?
   a. Forgets to turn in her homework, does not follow directions, cannot stay in her assigned seat in class, and is always talking excessively and inappropriately
   b. Is withdrawn in social contexts but energetic and engaging with her family
   c. Is stubborn, resistant to directions, and unwilling to negotiate
   d. Shows cruelty to animals, callousness, and lack of guilt and remorse

8. Jeremy, a 9-year-old with ADHD, has been placed on the stimulant methylphenidate (Ritalin, Concerta). You will know that your teaching has been effective when his parents state:
   a. "Jeremy will have an effect from this drug in about 2 weeks."
   b. "Jeremy may have some side effects, like insomnia, headache, or stomachache, but they are rare."
   c. "We'll bring Jeremy in every week to get his blood levels drawn."
   d. "Jeremy knows that he only needs to take this medication once every 12 hours."

9. Susan's parents have begun a program of therapy that includes giving Susan a token each time she follows directions. The following theoretical framework provides the background for such a program:
   a. behavioral theory.
   b. psychodynamic theory.
   c. systems theory.
   d. token economy theory.

10. John has become bored with his PlayStation, which had been his positive reward for cleaning his room. The most effective intervention with John at this time would be to
    a. tell John that he no longer has to clean his room in order to play.
    b. let John choose another reward that would be more fun.
    c. tell John that he has to use the PlayStation anyway, because it was expensive.
    d. reinforce to John that he selected the PlayStation, and he needs to stick with it.

CHAPTER 30

Working With Older Adults

Age 65 has arbitrarily become the point at which a person is considered old. To be more precise about the relationship between age and needs, the National Institute of Aging has defined chronological categories of the young old (ages 65 to 74 years), the middle old (ages 75 to 84 years), the old old (ages 85 to 94 years), and the elite old (ages 95 and older). Tasks of aging include conserving strength and resources as necessary and adapting to changes and losses that accompany the normal aging process. Changes and issues that most older adults confront include retirement, relocation, and bereavement.

Effective communication with older adults is one of the most important nursing interventions. Nurses will need to use specific techniques for those who have a hearing, visual, or cognitive deficit or display aggressive tendencies as a result of their condition. They also must avoid using any forms of degrading terminology. Approximately 25% of older adults in the community and more than 50% of those in nursing homes have symptoms of mental illness. Identifying and treating mental disorders in the older population is challenging because healthcare providers may confuse signs of normal aging with problems in mental functioning or may misdiagnose physical problems as mental illness.

Nurses must understand that the presentation of several psychiatric disorders can differ in older adults compared with the general population. A comprehensive assessment is vital. When administering and monitoring psychopharmacotherapy to older adults, nurses must handle issues involving adjustments in method of administration, polypharmacy, age-related differences in pharmacokinetics and pharmacodynamics, and the increased possibility of adverse and side effects.

Areas of mental health promotion for nurses to address when working with older adults include maintaining adequate nutrition and fluids, engaging in mental and physical activities, and ensuring adequate support systems.

LEARNING OBJECTIVES

After completing the exercises in this workbook, and studying the corresponding chapter in the textbook, the student will be able to:

- Identify different categories of older adults based on chronological age.

- Describe how sociocultural issues influence mental health.

- Explain why communication is so important for nurses working with older adults.

- Discuss attitudes that many in society hold toward older people.

- Discuss common geropsychiatric diagnoses and related nursing interventions.

- Evaluate important considerations related to the use of psychotropic medications in older adults.

- Discuss the nurse's role when caring for older people with mental or behavioral problems.

- Identify means to promote mental health and positive adaptation to aging for older clients.

KEY TERMS

Elite old: A chronological category used to designate those 95 years of age or older.

Middle old: A chronological category used to designate those 75 to 84 years of age.

Old old: A chronological category used to designate those 85 to 94 years of age.

Polypharmacy: Use of many drugs simultaneously by the same client.

Young old: A chronological category used to designate those 65 to 74 years of age.

Chapter Outline

DEMOGRAPHICS OF AGING AND FUTURE TRENDS
PSYCHOSOCIAL ISSUES AND INFLUENCES
Retirement
Relocation
Bereavement
Spirituality
Issues Related to Ethnicity and Language Barriers
COMMUNICATING EFFECTIVELY WITH OLDER ADULTS
Techniques
Terminology
ISSUES RELATED TO OLDER CLIENTS WITH PSYCHIATRIC DISORDERS

KEY TOPICS

Demographics of aging and future trends: Psychosocial issues (retirement, relocation, bereavement, spirituality, ethnicity and language barriers)

Communicating with older adults: Techniques, terminology

Issues related to older clients with psychiatric disorders: Ageism, myths, and prejudice; care settings; disorders; treatment

Promoting mental health and wellness in older adults: Nutrition, fluids, mental and physical activities; support systems

■ Exercises

CASE STUDY EXERCISE

Luther W. (nicknamed "Whit"), age 76, comes to his nurse practitioner with a complaint of weight loss of 45 lb over the past 6 months. Upon assessment, the nurse discovers that Whit's wife, Miriam, passed away 3 months ago secondary to kidney failure. She had become increasingly ill over the past 16 months and required intensive home care management, which had been done exclusively by Whit. Immediately following Miriam's death, Whit moved into the home of his youngest son, where he has a room for himself with ample space, including a small patio. Whit's son and daughter-in-law and their two children are his major source of support, in addition to another son in the area and a daughter who lives 8 hours away.

On interview, Whit states that his son and daughter have been urging him to go to his physician because of his weight loss, lack of appetite, difficulty sleeping, frequent tearfulness, and withdrawal. Whit is a Mason and had been very active in his local Lodge until about 6 months ago, when caring for his wife limited his ability to get to meetings. Whit denies suicidal ideation but admits that he has thought about death and dying a great deal since Miriam's death.

1. Conduct a comprehensive assessment of Whit, and delineate areas in which you have information and need more information.

2. What are Whit's current symptoms that may point to the possibility of a depressive episode? What else do you need to know to assess him for depression?

3. Discuss life events that may be precipitating Whit's current depression.

Whit is placed on Paxil, 20 mg q.d., by the physician. He reports that he has never been depressed before in his life and doesn't really think he needs the medication but is willing to try it.

4. What type of medication is Paxil? What are its mechanism of action, side effects, and target symptoms?

5. What will you include in client education about Paxil for Whit? What should he watch for, if anything?

After 3 weeks on Paxil, Whit reports that his appetite has improved, he has gained 3 lb, and he is now sleeping through most nights without awakening. His son reports that his father seems to be "in a much better mood, and is beginning to get up and around more during the day." Although Whit is often tearful if talking about his wife, Miriam, he is not crying off and on during the day like before.

6. What are goals for promoting Whit's general health.

7. How might you help Whit's son and his wife to care for themselves as they take on their roles as primary caretakers?

CRITICAL THINKING AND SELF-EVALUATION EXERCISES

1. Aging often brings losses and changes that come in large numbers over small amounts of time. Have you ever experienced a time in your life when you

have had a number of changes over a short time period? What was that like for you? Describe what helped you as you went through this period.

2. Whit is an actual older adult who lives in Florida. He welcomes you to visit his personal website (http://home.earthlink.net/~mijltwsr/) to learn more about his life and history.

■ NCLEX-Style Exam Questions

1. Age 65 has arbitrarily become designated as the point at which Americans are considered "old." This may be due to the fact that

   a. most people have to stop working at this age because they can no longer do their jobs.

   b. this is the age when Social Security and Medicare benefits become available.

   c. this is the age at which the body experiences physiological changes sufficient to affect functioning.

   d. most people feel older and begin to use the terminology of "old person" at age 65.

2. The National Institute of Aging has defined new chronological categories that now include

   a. elite old (95 years or older).

   b. morbidly old (99 years or older).

   c. middle-age older (45 to 55 years).

   d. elderly old (65 to 85 years).

3. In regard to developmental stages, which of the following is true about older age?

   a. The individual completes personal developmental stages prior to age 65.

   b. Individuals no longer go through formal developmental stages when they are older.

   c. Old age is a period of continued growth and development with its own tasks.

   d. If an individual never completed a specific developmental task, he or she may easily do so once he or she is elderly.

4. Maggie Smith is an 80-year-old white woman who says to her African American nurse, "Honey, I'd rather not have you bathe me. I want a white girl." The most therapeutic nursing intervention for this RN would be:

   a. "Mrs. Smith, I understand your feelings, but that is not possible. Can you talk about why you feel this way?"

   b. "Maggie, it's too bad that you don't want me to bathe you. We have no one else here who can do it."

   c. "Oh, Maggie, stop with your complaining. I'm doing your bath, and that's that."

   d. "Mrs. Smith, I wonder why you're saying that. Is there something about me that you don't like?"

5. Epidemiological studies have shown that the incidence of older adults in nursing homes who have symptoms of mental illness is

   a. around 90%.

   b. around 10%.

   c. around 5%.

   d. around 50%.

6. One of the biggest reasons older adults do not receive treatment for psychiatric disorders is that

   a. disease-related psychiatric symptoms are often misinterpreted as "normal" aging signs.

   b. they are ignored, even when they have the most disturbing symptoms.

   c. older adults often act confused and are thus categorized that way.

   d. aging individuals often have symptoms of depression and anxiety anyway, so these are normal symptoms for that age group.

7. One way in which the expression of depressive symptoms in older adults may differ from the presentation in young adults is

   a. older adults may somatize, or discuss their depressive symptoms in terms of physical symptoms or aches/pains.

   b. older adults tend to hold all their feelings in, whereas younger adults do not.

   c. older adults remain close to their families and thus become depressed over daily family issues, whereas younger adults often leave their families of origin.

   d. older adults may appear less suicidal than a younger adult who is depressed.

8. When using psychotropic medications in older adults, which of the following is true?

   a. Older adults often need more medication, because their livers do not metabolize as much of the drug as compared with younger people.

   b. Older adults need smaller doses of the same medication and become toxic more quickly than do younger adults.

c. Older adults should rarely be given psychotropic medications unless they are suicidal.

d. Older adults often do not understand why they are receiving psychotropic medications.

9. Madge Jones is an 88-year-old African American woman in a nursing home. She is alert and is frequently seen talking and laughing with other clients. Over a period of a few days, you notice that she has become quiet, is disoriented, and is running a low-grade fever. Which of the following might you suspect first?

a. She may be becoming demented.

b. She may have a urinary tract infection.

c. She may be depressed.

d. She may be experiencing delirium.

10. Educating new nurses regarding ageism would be considered successful if a new RN graduate is heard to say

a. "Since the elderly have so many losses and changes, it is normal to expect them to have a major depressive episode at some point during their elderly years."

b. "Elderly persons are so wise and expert about everything life has to offer."

c. "It is critical to treat each elderly person as an individual and to be sure to understand their own life story and events that are affecting them during their older years."

d. "Elderly people should be treated with kindness because they do not have many years left."

Answer Key

Chapter 1

GENERAL MATCHING

1. j
2. c
3. b
4. g
5. a
6. i
7. d
8. h
9. e
10. f

DSM-IV-TR MATCHING

a. 3
b. 1
c. 2
d. 2
e. 4
f. 5
g. 1
h. 1

COMPLETION

1. passive–aggressive
2. altruistic
3. suicide
4. culturally competent
5. basic

NCLEX-STYLE EXAM QUESTIONS

1. b
2. c
3. d
4. a
5. b
6. a
7. b
8. b
9. a
10. b

Chapter 2

MATCHING

1. c
2. i
3. a
4. f
5. d
6. b
7. h
8. g
9. e
10. j

SHORT ANSWER

1. second hit
2. Learning; memory
3. circadian rhythm
4. Psychoneuroimmunology
5. neurotransmitters
6. brain stem; vital signs, respirations, sleep and wakeful-ness, visual and auditory reflexes
7. critical period
8. Reactive; adaptive
9. transcription; translation
10. concordance rate

DIAGRAM LABELING

Brain Structures

1. Central sulcus
2. Parietal lobe
3. Occipital lobe
4. Cerebellum
5. Spinal cord
6. Medulla oblongata
7. Pons
8. Midbrain
9. Temporal lobe
10. Lateral sulcus
11. Frontal lobe
12. Gyri

Brain Functions

1. Motor cortex
2. Sensory area (pain, touch, etc.)
3. Visual interpretation area
4. Visual receiving area
5. Auditory interpretation area
6. Auditory receiving area
7. Motor speech
8. Written speech

NCLEX-STYLE EXAM QUESTIONS

1. a
2. a
3. b
4. d
5. d
6. a
7. c
8. b
9. b
10. c

Chapter 3

MATCHING

1. b
2. h
3. g
4. j
5. c

6. e
7. d
8. f
9. i
10. a

COMPLETION

1. psychodynamic
2. theory
3. hypothesis
4. id; ego; superego
5. countertransference
6. respondent conditioning; operant conditioning
7. positive
8. modeling
9. cognitive restructuring
10. risk factors

NCLEX-STYLE EXAM QUESTIONS

1. c
2. a
3. a
4. d
5. a
6. b
7. c
8. d
9. d
10. a

Chapter 4

MATCHING

1. c
2. g
3. j
4. d
5. f
6. h
7. b
8. e
9. k
10. a
11. i

SHORT ANSWER

1. Social responding
   a. Purpose: Engaging in superficial conversation that is not client-centered
   b. Example:
      Client: "I am happy to finally be going to group today."
      Nurse: "The room it is held in is really sunny."
2. Closed-ended questions
   a. Purpose: Questions that elicit a "yes" or "no" answer
   b. Example: "Do you know what that medication is for?"

3. Changing the subject
   a. Purpose: Introducing an unrelated or peripherally related topic
   b. Example:
      Client: "I used cocaine just before I came into the unit today."
      Nurse: "Well, before that, did you have a good time at the game?"
4. Belittling
   a. Purpose: Discounting client's feelings or making comparisons that imply her problems are smaller than she perceives
   b. Example:
      Client: "I am so upset that I'm in here and not able to work."
      Nurse: "Well, don't worry; a lot of people in here will never be able to go back to work. At least you'll be able to someday."
5. Making stereotyped comments
   a. Purpose: Offering platitudes or wise sayings that seem automatic or contrived.
   b. Example:
      Client: "My cancer has now spread to my kidneys."
      Nurse: "Now, try and look on the bright side—there's always hope for a cure!"
6. False reassurance
   a. Purpose: Attempting to cheer the client up by suggesting there is no real problem.
   b. Example:
      Client: "I can't believe I am so depressed that I ended up in here."
      Nurse: "Not to worry. You'll be happy and back to work in no time."
7. Moralizing
   a. Purpose: Passing judgment by imposing one's own values on the client and implying that his or her way of thinking is wrong
   b. Example:
      Client: "I have just discovered that I am gay."
      Nurse: "I think you should pray about that, because you can often turn yourself around with enough support."
8. Interpreting
   a. Purpose: Making intrusive comments in an attempt to psychoanalyze clients
   b. Example:
      Client: "I just don't want to go home on a day pass."
      Nurse: "I think you are avoiding painful feelings by not confronting your anger at your parents."
9. Advising
   a. Purpose: Making specific suggestions instead of offering information and asking clients what they think might work
   b. Example:
      Client: "I am so upset that my husband has not visited me."
      Nurse: "You need to call him up and tell him you need to see him."

10. Challenging
    a. Purpose: Denying the client's perceptions
    b. Example:
       Client: "None of the staff here like me."
       Nurse: "What about the party yesterday? I saw several staff talking and laughing with you."
11. Defending
    a. Purpose: Arguing or justifying your position rather than attempting to hear the client's concerns
    b. Example:
       Client: "I am never able to get my shaving stuff when I need it."
       Nurse: "Well, I'm sorry, but we are really busy and you will just have to deal with it."

CORRECT THE FALSE STATEMENTS

1. Despite the incredible developments in technology that hold promise for treatment of psychiatric disorders, the primary medium through which all psychiatric care is provided is still the *therapeutic relationship*.
2. *Confidentiality* is a component of trust, and includes the right for clients to conceal that they are receiving treatment for a mental health problem.
3. *Caring* consists of three primary behaviors: giving of the self, meeting the client's needs in a timely manner, and providing comfort measures for clients and their families.
4. *Empathy* involves listening carefully, being in tune with what clients are saying, and having insight into the meaning of their thoughts, feelings, and behaviors.
5. The nurse exhibits a *judgmental attitude* when she states, "I think Joan should just pull herself up by her bootstraps; she isn't even trying to help herself."

CASE STUDY: NURSING PROCESS EXERCISE

Jamie is a *24-year-old schoolteacher* who is admitted to the psychiatric unit by a police officer. After *"binge drinking" last night,* which resulted in her *passing out,* she awoke with a *severe anxiety attack* because she *did not know where she was.* She *has experienced mild "panic attacks" (as she describes them) in the past,* but this one is *worse than any before.* It appeared to Jamie *that perhaps she had been raped,* which brought back *memories of an experience of abuse at the age of 12.* She was *aching all over,* was *undressed,* and began to *hear a radio playing in her head.* She dialed 911 on a phone in the room and was picked up by a police officer, who brought her to the emergency department. She was *screened for rape* in the ED, but there was *no evidence of rape.*

When she arrives on your unit, Jamie is *disheveled* and states very anxiously that the *radio noise in her head "just won't stop!"* She is *shaking,* is *sweating mildly,* and complains of a *racing heartbeat* with *difficulty breathing.* When you introduce yourself to Jamie, *she seems to ignore you, or seems not to even hear you speaking.*

To the Student: In this chapter of the Study Guide, a Nursing Care Planning Worksheet is completed as an example of how the student should complete the worksheets. See page 158. In future chapters, the student will be asked to complete the worksheet, but answers will not be provided. The student should refer to the appropriate chapter in the textbook to guide the selection of nursing diagnoses, goals, and interventions for specific client difficulties.

NCLEX-STYLE EXAM QUESTIONS

1. b
2. d
3. b
4. b
5. b
6. d
7. a
8. d
9. d
10. b

Chapter 5

GENERAL MATCHING

1. b
2. e
3. j
4. a
5. g
6. i
7. h
8. c
9. f
10. d

SOCIOCULTURAL GROUP MATCHING

1. b
2. d
3. a
4. c

SHORT ANSWER

1. Cross-Cultural Understanding
   a. Knowledge about how and why people of different cultures behave in certain ways
   b. You ask a friend who is of a different culture to talk with you about her/his values, beliefs, and cultural influences on behavior.
2. Intercultural Communication
   a. Communication techniques that vary between/among cultures, such as openness, self-disclosure, emotional expression, insight, and talkativeness
   b. You spend additional time with a client who is from a different culture than your own to ensure that you are providing culturally competent care.
3. Facilitation Skills
   a. Focuses on conflict resolution and ability to negotiate interactions that may not be consistent with your own culture
   b. You work with the client to understand the cultural beliefs about conflict and negotiation in his/her own culture in order to work within those cultural norms.

NURSING PROCESS WORKSHEET[1]

Health Problem (Title)

Anxiety

Related to

↓

Etiology (Related Factors)

Prior evening of "binge drinking", awakening in a foreign place, and re-experiencing of a past trauma

Evidenced by

↓

**Signs and Symptoms
(Defining Characteristics)**

Hearing radio noise in head, shaking, sweating, tachycardia, tachypnea, inability to concentrate

Client Goal*

Jamie will experience a reduction in symtoms of anxiety within the next 8 hours.

Nursing Interventions**

1. Continue to assess symptoms of anxiety, including withdrawal signs
2. Monitor Vital Signs and Hydration
3. Provide low stimulus environment
4. Administer medications as ordered
5. Provide brief, frequent contacts to build trust

Evaluative Statement

Jamie has become calmer during the past 8 hours, and reports no shaking, sweating, or palpitations. She is able to attend to directions and is beginning to talk about her experience.

[1]Refer to textbook, Chapter 6, for more information about Care Planning.

*More than one client goal may be appropriate. For this exercise, choose one client goal that demonstrates a direct resolution of the client problem identified in the nursing diagnosis.

**Be sure you are able to list the scientific rationale for each nursing intervention you order.

4. Flexibility
   a. The ability to embrace change by modifying expectations, readjusting old norms and stereotypes, and trying new behaviors
   b. You work with a client and her family in order to provide time and space to conduct spiritual ceremonies for healing.

NCLEX-STYLE EXAM QUESTIONS
1. b
2. b
3. b
4. a
5. d
6. a
7. b
8. a
9. b
10. a

Chapter 6

MATCHING, PART A
1. b
2. a
3. c
4. e
5. i
6. h
7. f
8. j
9. g
10. k
11. d

MATCHING, PART B
1. d
2. h
3. j
4. a
5. e
6. i
7. g
8. c
9. e
10. k
11. g

NCLEX-STYLE EXAM QUESTIONS
1. c
2. a
3. d
4. a
5. c
6. a
7. d
8. b
9. d
10. b

Chapter 7

MATCHING
1. d
2. a
3. i
4. e
5. b
6. c
7. f
8. g
9. h
10. j

NCLEX-STYLE EXAM QUESTIONS
1. c
2. b
3. c
4. a
5. a
6. b
7. d
8. a
9. c
10. c

Chapter 8

MATCHING
1. b
2. c
3. a
4. f
5. h
6. g
7. f
8. e
9. d
10. i

CASE STUDY
1. The three components of the cognitive triad, and supporting data, are as follows:
   a. Negative view of self: John's statement that he is a "horrible person"
   b. Negative view of the world: His statements that "my entire world is upside down" and "It seems that nothing ever goes my way."
   c. Negative view of the future: "His statement that "I really can't see a future for myself."
2. Other theories that might be chosen: behavioral, cognitive, rational-emotive, choice.

NCLEX-STYLE EXAM QUESTIONS
1. c
2. b
3. d
4. c
5. b

6. c
7. b
8. a
9. a
10. d

Chapter 9

MATCHING
1. d
2. e
3. g
4. i
5. a
6. h
7. b
8. f
9. c
10. j

NCLEX-STYLE EXAM QUESTIONS
1. c
2. d
3. d
4. a
5. a
6. a
7. c
8. b
9. b
10. b

Chapter 10

MATCHING
1. b
2. a
3. f
4. c
5. e
6. h
7. i
8. d
9. j
10. g

NCLEX-STYLE EXAM QUESTIONS
1. a
2. d
3. b
4. c
5. c
6. b
7. d
8. b
9. c
10. b

Chapter 11

MATCHING
1. g
2. j
3. h
4. b
5. i
6. d
7. a
8. c
9. f
10. e

CORRECT THE FALSE STATEMENTS
1. Currently, *Poland* has the highest incarceration rate in the Western world.
2. Forensic clients often demonstrate poor judgment, *limited but available family support,* limited reasoning abilities, and exceptionally high levels of *anxiety* disorders.
3. *Instrumental* violence is associated with group membership and is usually done for revenge or retaliation for a perceived wrong.
4. Forensic psychiatric nurses are often *secure in their roles* and have dual obligations: one of social necessity and social good and one *of maintaining safety in the jail facility.*
5. In forensic settings, the incidence of self-violence and suicide is much *lower* than in the general population because of the extreme, 24-hour monitoring systems in place.
6. The active crisis state is *long-term,* usually lasting *at least 3 months.*
7. The *first* phase of a crisis is marked by anxiety caused by the failure of usual coping mechanisms; the *second* phase includes anxiety in response to a trauma; the *third* phase involves the inadequacy of the person's inner resources and supports; and the *fourth* is marked by escalating anxiety.
8. Melody was in a building when the roof caved in next to her. She becomes depressed and anxious, reflecting the onset of a *developmental* crisis.
9. Crisis intervention differs from traditional therapies in that it focuses more on the *individual's past experiences and their relationship to current events.*
10. *Black* men are the primary group that can be found in homeless shelters, although *white couples are increasingly being found in shelters in large cities.*
11. Research has shown that the homeless mentally ill account for *85%* of the homeless population, and that over *70%* of the total homeless population demonstrate symptoms of *anxiety.*
12. Common contributing factors to homelessness include lack of mental health care, *poor work ethics, anergia,* inadequate supportive housing, *avolition,* and the stigma and discrimination associated with mental illness.
13. Major goals for a homeless mentally ill person include: Client will satisfy physical needs and remain safe; *Client will engage in educational opportunities to*

establish experience for employment; Client will identify and use psychosocial supports; *Client will report to therapist every 2 weeks, minimally.*

NCLEX-STYLE EXAM QUESTIONS
1. d
2. d
3. a
4. a
5. a
6. a
7. c
8. d
9. a
10. b

Chapter 12

MATCHING
1. g
2. d
3. j
4. a
5. h
6. b
7. i
8. e
9. c
10. f

NCLEX-STYLE EXAM QUESTIONS
1. b
2. c
3. b
4. c
5. c
6. b
7. c
8. b
9. a
10. c

Chapter 13

SENTENCE COMPLETION
1. Spirituality
2. Religion
3. Spiritual; health
4. Values
5. chaplain

CORRECT THE FALSE STATEMENTS
1. F
2. T
3. T
4. F
5. F

NCLEX-STYLE EXAM QUESTIONS
1. c
2. d
3. d
4. b
5. a
6. c
7. a
8. a
9. a
10. a

Chapter 14

MATCHING
1. a
2. d
3. e
4. a
5. d
6. e
7. b
8. d
9. a
10. c
11. a
12. e
13. e
14. b
15. c
16. b
17. e
18. c

NCLEX-STYLE EXAM QUESTIONS
1. b
2. c
3. b
4. b
5. c
6. a
7. d
8. a
9. c
10. a

Chapter 15

MATCHING
1. b
2. i
3. e
4. d
5. j
6. h
7. c
8. f
9. a
10. g

NCLEX-STYLE EXAM QUESTIONS

1. a
2. a
3. c
4. c
5. b
6. c
7. d
8. a
9. a
10. b

Chapter 16

MATCHING

1. e
2. a
3. b
4. d
5. c

SHORT ANSWER

1. Types of services included under the umbrella of home health care services are medical, social work, psychological services; chemical dependency counselors; physical therapy; occupational and vocational therapy; speech and recreational therapy; dental and pharmacy services.
2. Goals of behavioral health home care are to teaching problem solving, stress reduction, and coping skills to clients and family members or caregivers; providing respite and community resources to family members and caregivers; educating clients and their family member/caregiver about mental illness and wellness, medications, relapse prevention, and communication skills; and coordinating and integrating the client's medical, social, spiritual, vocational, and other services.
3. Critical indicators of the need for behavioral health home care are mental health status changes or impairments; history of frequent hospitalizations, recurrent episodes of mental illness, or both; multiple functional limitations; changes in health status, material welfare, home environment, family, social support network, behavioral health functioning, motivation, leisure time or diversionary activities; needs for health or medication teaching; anticipatory guidance, psychiatric crisis or emergency.

CORRECT THE FALSE STATEMENTS

1. Home care has been delivered in the United States since the *1950s.*
2. It was not until *the first National Psychiatric Home Care Conference was held in 1994* that nurses began to hold conferences around behavioral health care.
3. Two goals of home health care are to gain, regain, maintain, or restore the client's optimal state of health and independence and *minimize and rehabilitate the effects of illness before or after institutionalization.*

4. A behavioral health clinical nurse specialist is an *MSN-prepared psychiatric nurse* who has had specialized education for assessment and intervention skills and is ANA certified in *adult psychiatric and mental health nursing.*
5. In accordance with the *ANA Standards of Home Health Nursing Practice,* the behavioral health home care nurse assesses the client and family.

NCLEX-STYLE EXAM QUESTIONS

1. c
2. c
3. a
4. c
5. d
6. a
7. a
8. d
9. b
10. a

Chapter 17

MATCHING

1. f
2. b
3. g
4. e
5. c
6. h
7. a
8. j
9. d
10. i

NCLEX-STYLE EXAM QUESTIONS

1. a
2. b
3. a
4. a
5. a
6. b
7. a
8. a
9. b
10. c

Chapter 18

CASE STUDY ANSWERS

The case study in this chapter is from the practice of a psychiatric–mental health advanced practice nurse. It is an actual clinical case with a client who suffers from an anxiety disorder. The case study poses several clinical situations in which there is usually more than one correct answer, given the clinical facts. Therefore, for case study answers, the student is encouraged to use the textbook and discussion with faculty and peers to determine appropriate care strategies, given the clinical scenario presented, and to provide a rationale for the choices made.

NCLEX-STYLE EXAM QUESTIONS
1. b
2. d
3. c
4. b
5. d
6. a
7. a
8. a
9. a
10. c

Chapter 19

CASE STUDY ANSWERS
The case study in this chapter is from the practice of a psychiatric–mental health advanced practice nurse. The case study poses several clinical situations in which there is usually more than one correct answer, given the clinical facts. Therefore, for case study answers, the student is encouraged to use the textbook and discussion with faculty and peers to determine appropriate care strategies, given the clinical scenario presented, and to provide a rationale for the choices made.

NCLEX-STYLE EXAM QUESTIONS
1. d
2. a
3. a
4. a
5. b
6. d
7. c
8. d
9. c
10. d

Chapter 20

CASE STUDY ANSWERS
The case study in this chapter is from the practice of a psychiatric–mental health advanced practice nurse. The case study poses several clinical situations in which there is usually more than one correct answer, given the clinical facts. Therefore, for case study answers, the student is encouraged to use the textbook and discussion with faculty and peers to determine appropriate care strategies, given the clinical scenario presented, and to provide a rationale for the choices made.

NCLEX-STYLE EXAM QUESTIONS
1. b
2. a

3. d
4. d
5. a
6. d
7. a
8. b
9. d
10. d

Chapter 21

CASE STUDY ANSWERS
The case study in this chapter is from the practice of a psychiatric–mental health advanced practice nurse. The case study poses several clinical situations in which there is usually more than one correct answer, given the clinical facts. Therefore, for case study answers, the student is encouraged to use the textbook and discussion with faculty and peers to determine appropriate care strategies, given the clinical scenario presented, and to provide a rationale for the choices made.

NCLEX-STYLE EXAM QUESTIONS
1. c
2. d
3. d
4. a
5. c
6. a
7. d
8. b
9. a
10. d

Chapter 22

CASE STUDY ANSWERS
The case study in this chapter is from the practice of a psychiatric–mental health advanced practice nurse. The case study poses several clinical situations in which there is usually more than one correct answer, given the clinical facts. Therefore, for case study answers, the student is encouraged to use the textbook and discussion with faculty and peers to determine appropriate care strategies, given the clinical scenario presented, and to provide a rationale for the choices made.

NCLEX-STYLE EXAM QUESTIONS
1. d
2. b
3. a
4. a
5. d
6. c
7. b
8. a
9. c
10. d

Chapter 23

CASE STUDY ANSWERS

The case study in this chapter is from the practice of a psychiatric–mental health advanced practice nurse. The case study poses several clinical situations in which there is usually more than one correct answer, given the clinical facts. Therefore, for case study answers, the student is encouraged to use the textbook and discussion with faculty and peers to determine appropriate care strategies, given the clinical scenario presented, and to provide a rationale for the choices made.

NCLEX-STYLE EXAM QUESTIONS

1. a
2. c
3. d
4. a
5. b
6. a
7. d
8. a
9. d
10. d

Chapter 24

CASE STUDY ANSWERS

The case study in this chapter is from the practice of a psychiatric–mental health advanced practice nurse. The case study poses several clinical situations in which there is usually more than one correct answer, given the clinical facts. Therefore, for case study answers, the student is encouraged to use the textbook and discussion with faculty and peers to determine appropriate care strategies, given the clinical scenario presented, and to provide a rationale for the choices made.

NCLEX-STYLE EXAM QUESTIONS

1. a
2. c
3. c
4. b
5. b
6. d
7. a
8. b
9. a
10. d

Chapter 25

CASE STUDY ANSWERS

The case study in this chapter is from the practice of a psychiatric–mental health advanced practice nurse. The case study poses several clinical situations in which there is

usually more than one correct answer, given the clinical facts. Therefore, for case study answers, the student is encouraged to use the textbook and discussion with faculty and peers to determine appropriate care strategies, given the clinical scenario presented, and to provide a rationale for the choices made.

NCLEX-STYLE EXAM QUESTIONS

1. a
2. b
3. c
4. c
5. c
6. c
7. a
8. a
9. c
10. a

Chapter 26

CASE STUDY ANSWERS

The case study in this chapter is from the practice of a psychiatric–mental health advanced practice nurse. The case study poses several clinical situations in which there is usually more than one correct answer, given the clinical facts. Therefore, for case study answers, the student is encouraged to use the textbook and discussion with faculty and peers to determine appropriate care strategies, given the clinical scenario presented, and to provide a rationale for the choices made.

NCLEX-STYLE EXAM QUESTIONS

1. a
2. d
3. b
4. c
5. d
6. b
7. b
8. a
9. a
10. c

Chapter 27

CASE STUDY ANSWERS

The case study in this chapter is from the practice of a psychiatric–mental health advanced practice nurse. The case study poses several clinical situations in which there is usually more than one correct answer, given the clinical facts. Therefore, for case study answers, the student is encouraged to use the textbook and discussion with faculty and peers to determine appropriate care strategies, given the clinical scenario presented, and to provide a rationale for the choices made.

NCLEX-STYLE EXAM QUESTIONS
1. c
2. a
3. d
4. b
5. b
6. c
7. c
8. b
9. c
10. a

Chapter 28

CASE STUDY ANSWERS

The case study in this chapter is from the practice of a psychiatric–mental health advanced practice nurse. The case study poses several clinical situations in which there is usually more than one correct answer, given the clinical facts. Therefore, for case study answers, the student is encouraged to use the textbook and discussion with faculty and peers to determine appropriate care strategies, given the clinical scenario presented, and to provide a rationale for the choices made.

NCLEX-STYLE EXAM QUESTIONS
1. a
2. c
3. b
4. c
5. b
6. a
7. b
8. a
9. d
10. b

Chapter 29

CASE STUDY ANSWERS

The case study in this chapter is from the practice of a psychiatric–mental health advanced practice nurse. The case study poses several clinical situations in which there is usually more than one correct answer, given the clinical facts. Therefore, for case study answers, the student is encouraged to use the textbook and discussion with faculty and peers to determine appropriate care strategies, given the clinical scenario presented, and to provide a rationale for the choices made.

NCLEX-STYLE EXAM QUESTIONS
1. a
2. d
3. d
4. a
5. c
6. a
7. a
8. b
9. a
10. b

Chapter 30

CASE STUDY ANSWERS

The case study in this chapter is that of an actual older adult who is known to the author. Whit has undergone many of the usual experiences of loss, change, and aging. The case study poses several clinical situations in which there is usually more than one correct answer, given the clinical facts. Therefore, for case study answers, the student is encouraged to use the textbook and discussion with faculty and peers to determine appropriate care strategies, given the clinical scenario presented, and to provide a rationale for the choices made. The student is encouraged to visit Whit's personal website to learn more about his life.

NCLEX-STYLE EXAM QUESTIONS
1. b
2. a
3. c
4. a
5. d
6. a
7. a
8. b
9. b
10. c